Forget About Diets. You are a Food Addict

A recovered obese will teach you the proven 3+4 Method to achieve weight loss and maintain a healthy weight for life.

Rupert B. Carter

Acknowledgment

To my wife and son – my love, my life, my light.

ISBN: 978-0-9571961-5-5

Contents

Author Biography

If you ever thought you were alone with your weight struggles, finally Rupert B. Carter is here to tell you differently. As a recovered 'professional' obese person, he has hit rock bottom with his weight, and made it back to tell his tale.

"I have tried endless techniques and diets, and always ended up with the same results: Yo-yo dieting and gaining even more weight than I had before. My family gave up on me. Both my wife and son were always laughing every time I said, this time my diet was for real. They didn't trust me, for a good reason. I never stick to any diet. Never!".

Both Rupert's parents were obese, and he was raised believing that being a bit overweight wasn't a big deal. Food was a cornerstone of comfort and escape. Celebrations always involved the wrong kinds of food, because in those days, people didn't really know any better.

Rupert didn't think twice about eating as much pizza, white bread, ice creams, cookies, chocolates and as much sugar-loaded coffee as he wanted. However, ultimately this left him feeling unhealthy, unfit, and ashamed of his lack of control. Like many of us do, he took his failure to regulate his weight as an indication that he was weak, and somehow broken.

That was before he created the 3+4 Method that has helped him, and many others, turn this age-old story around. After over 30 years of yo-yo diets, this new way of thinking has helped him lose weight and keep it off for the last five years.

His breakthrough came when he realized he was a food addict. Once he could admit his addiction, it opened a vast range of possibilities for change on all levels: mental, emotional, physical, and in the rest of his life.

By sharing his story, he hopes to help others on the same journey to both realize and deal with their own food addiction. His practical approach, loaded with tools, exercise, and strategies, is the ultimate guide to finally getting control of the weight that perhaps you had given up on changing before now.

Introduction

Does your extra weight leave you feeling ugly and ashamed?

Are you sick of people coming up to you and oversharing their unwanted opinions about weight and diets? Maybe, you have even started avoiding social gatherings as a result? And don't get me started on the occasional sad, binge eating, especially late at night in front of the TV, or when you are feeling bad, lonely, or bored.

Listen up!

It does not have to be this way.

Food addiction has been on the rise for decades, and weight-related deaths, illnesses, mental and social dysfunctions, and the base cost to the nation is climbing exponentially. If you have any doubt that you are a food addict, you will find clarity here. Maybe, you are simply on the slippery slope to becoming a full-blown food addict. If you:

- eat when you feel mad, bad, sad, or anxious.
- eat when you don't feel hungry.
- eat when you feel bored or restless.
- eat to soothe yourself.
- eat until you feel stuffed, or even ill.

Then there is a problem.

Sure, there are plenty of diet pills, diet gurus, and a million people offering their tried-and-tested methods to lose weight.

It's a multi-billion-dollar industry these days. What is different here is that this book takes a completely holistic and practical view of human nature, the science of eating, and of the food addiction crisis sweeping the globe. It combines key learning from every health and lifestyle modality that can be used to address this challenge. And it is based on personal experience, not just theory.

There is not one magic pill that will fix it. It takes a lot of small (and some big) steps, and it takes time. You will need to learn new coping skills, and build focus, resilience, and self-discipline. All the tools you need to do so are given to you here.

This is a journey you will take that will bring everything you need to know about food challenges, and self-care, together in a step-by-step method that leaves no stone unturned.

Your real weight-loss answers are, truly, within these pages.

Sharing my journey with you

The laughter hurt. It hurt way more than anyone realized.

I gazed down at the salad I had ordered. The greens were piled high, and it was dotted with croutons and drizzled with a creamy dressing. It was definitely not the burger and fries I had wanted to order. I was trying to lose weight, again.

This wasn't the first time.

My friends didn't mean to be cruel. The laughter was half good-natured, and half in disbelief that I had ordered a salad. They had seen this story play out so many times before. They felt sorry for me.

My face and ears burned with shame. I could hear the grating metal legs of my chair on the concrete of the restaurant floor, as I pushed it back, mumbled some excuse, and walked out. I felt like an idiot but couldn't sit there another second.

I needed some air. I needed a break. Anger, frustration, and pain washed through me in cycles.

"Why am I even bothering?"

I had been down this road so many times before. Inspired by a new diet, or health regimen, I would start out on a high that soon became another low, as the weight fell off and then just piled back on again. Each time I felt worse. Often, I put back even more weight than before. Those people who lost all that weight, and kept it off, seemed like they lived in another land. They looked great in their slick gym gear, smiling while they chugged their smoothies, and I just couldn't relate to them. They had something I didn't.

Was it motivation? Was it resilience? What was the secret? Why could they stick with it? Why did it work for them and not for me? It was so demotivating. It was so freaking hard. Did anyone realize how hard it was to go on a diet, cut out the carbs, eat healthy, and then just see all that effort backfire a few weeks, or even days, later?

Each time it happened, I lost more faith in myself as a person, and so did my friends and family. We all saw I couldn't stick to anything. If I couldn't follow through on what I ate, what else in life couldn't I get right? I felt that question deeply, and I could see it reflected in their eyes, too.

Then a still, small voice in my head stopped the negative mental rollercoaster.

"It's different this time. You know it is."

I went back into that restaurant, sat down, and sent back that salad. "Just the spinach, sesame seeds, and avocado, please. Hold the croutons and give me some dressing on the side." I smiled around at all my friends, and ate my salad, enjoying every bite. I knew something that they did not. Not yet! Not at that moment. They did see later, and some even had the character to apologize for not believing in me and supporting me like they should have. I couldn't blame them. Up until then, I really hadn't been handling things well. My failure had become so predictable it was boring, and a joke.

However, I had had a breakthrough that had suddenly made all the difference. I was a food addict! And until I dealt with my eating habits, just like any other addict would face their addictions, nothing I did was ever going to work long term.

This deep understanding had started to change my life from that pivotal AHA moment. It changed everything. How I looked at myself, and my eating, shifted. How I dealt with the problem needed a whole new approach.

Addiction, in any form, requires us to pull out the big guns. It is a horrible situation for the addict, and for those around them. It is harmful to the body, mind, and soul. And it hurts those around you, too.

The simple fact that my weight had resulted in skyrocketing blood pressure, that I was now pre-diabetic, and that my doctor was seriously concerned about my health was a big issue. I was obese. My health and life insurance were loaded. And I had been told several times that I was playing a life-and-death game that would ultimately result in my family losing me, earlier rather than later. Not only that, but my weight prevented us from doing stuff. I couldn't even take short walks with my son, let alone play any games with him. On the plane, I had to book two seats and huffed and puffed my way through life battling with things most people take for granted. Stuff like awkward chair sizes and the embarrassment of trying to find somewhere to sit that fits, like not even finding your size in a plus-size clothing store, or not being able to go on family outings. It meant that my addiction was hurting my family, too.

I had heard the same old things all my life. Does any of this sound like you?

- You have been yo-yo dieting for several years, decades, or even your whole life.
- You believe you can't lose weight because you don't have the willpower.
- You were taught that your problem is your calorie intake.
- You were taught a diet is the key to solve your weight problem.
- You quit your diet when you are sad.
- You quit your diet when you are happy and want to celebrate.
- You quit your diet when you are tired and want something quick.

- You quit your diet when you see that (extra-large) clothes are fitting better.
- You quit your diet when you are told that you have lost weight and look fabulous.
- You quit your diet when you want to avoid throwing away junk food.
- You quit your diet when you are at any social gatherings like birthdays, end of the year, Christmas, Thanksgiving, club night, dinner with friends, and movie night.
- You quit your diet when you are at home relaxing.
- You quit your diet when you find no health food in the fridge.
- You quit your diet when you get to Friday and over the weekend.
- You quit your diet when you eat out and every time someone else dining with you eats junk food.
- You believe you'll start your diet again on Monday, or in a few days' time.
- You buy junk food at the supermarket for your family. And then you are the one who ends up eating it.
- You struggle to say no to people offering you junk food.
- You always have plenty of pills to relieve heartburn, indigestion, and an upset stomach.
- You are truly concerned about your health issues or developing potentially obesity-related health issues—for

example, high cholesterol, coronary heart disease, type 2 diabetes, stroke, some types of cancer, hypertension, arthritis and joint problems, fertility problems, asthma, back pain, incontinence, gout, and sleep apnoea.

- Your jeans rip in the inner thighs.
- You are concerned your children will follow your example and become (or are) overweight.
- You are concerned about your family's future when you think you may die from obesity-related diseases.
- You have given up on your appearance and believe you will always be overweight.
- Your friends and family have given up on you. They believe you will never stick to any diet, nor reach a healthy weight ever again.
- You don't buy new clothes, because you believe you will lose weight and be able to use your small sizes very soon. That never happens, and you keep clothes from 10 years ago.
- You convince yourself you are not that fat, because your (extra-large) clothes are not that tight.
- Your family (including your children) constantly tells you that you need to lose weight.
- You were taught that everyone in your family must eat the same food at dinner time.
- You were taught you are overweight due to factors out of your control, such as metabolism or genes.

- You convince yourself you are eating unhealthy food as it is cheaper, faster, and you want to save money.
- You believe that you are on the right track because you choose 'light' junk food substitutes or stuff with 'diet' and 'zero' on the label.
- You wait for a perfect date, a particular event, or the right mood to start a diet.
- You think that you can be fat and healthy.
- You have convinced yourself that healthy food is not tasty, and you will not enjoy your diet.
- You have visited nutritionists, and nothing seemed to work.
- You have tried endless diets and are still waiting for the one that will change your life.
- You set weight loss as a key annual resolution every new year.
- You wish you could move on to other priority goals in your life, but you just need to get on top of the weight thing first.
- You experience guilt every time you eat junk food.
- You gained weight over many years and think it must just be your age.
- You have put on so much weight over a long period of time. How will you ever catch up, or lose all that?

If you answered yes to any of these things, you are on the right track reading this book. I was in your shoes. I kept trying and failing. I wanted to improve things, but I just didn't know what to do. My insight that I was a food addict changed that.

There is a lot of misleading advice from diet gurus and exercise experts out there. And yes, some of it works for some people, but not so far for you, right? If you saw yourself in the descriptions above, your answer may be a little different.

My real solution wasn't about trying some new diet or spending more time on a treadmill. To get to the root of the issue I had to do two things. I had to understand addiction better, such as how food and the brain and body interacted. I also had to understand what was triggering my addiction, such as what thoughts and feelings were driving me, and what pain I wasn't facing.

Because with any addiction, there is always pain underneath. That is what it is all about. Numbing the bad feelings. Food was my painkiller of choice, and over time, I needed more and more of it to get the same effect.

Understanding all of this has led to lasting change for me.

For quite some time, I have been fit, healthy, and at goal weight. This is not some get-thin-quick scheme, if that is what you were thinking. This takes work. And it takes the right kind of effort.

It means facing fears, unravelling pain, and digging deep into the past and present to release all the emotional and mental blocks an addict sits with. It means understanding that you can't do it alone. That you need support systems in place and loads of easy-to-use tools for those times when things get tough. And they do get tough.

It took me hitting my lowest point to finally see myself more clearly and to admit there was an addiction problem. And then

I needed to get really clear on why I wanted things to change. For me, there were a few things. I wanted the respect of my son, my wife, and my friends back. I wanted to be free of this inner pain that sat like a black lump in my life. This was finally important enough for me to drive me to action.

It was a steep learning curve. It took me a while, and it took a lot of courage. I want to share my journey with you. I believe that if I could have had someone share this stuff with me up front, it would have been a lot easier. I had to learn the hard way, and do a lot of research, trial-and-error effort, and all of this took me a lot longer.

I want to help others sitting in my situation. I want to take a little of the pain away, and give you hope, not only with my story, but also with practical know-how and tools that will help you create your own success story, too. I know you can do it because I did. And I know many who have also benefited from my learning already.

My 3+4 Method will help you achieve the best version of yourself through a healthy body and mind and, in this book, I will tell you how to do so in seven practical steps.

It includes three steps to raise self-awareness and remind you of who you are. And then another four steps to actually lose that weight, once and for all.

Some people love the quick and easy stuff, such as magical solutions with colorful dishes, inspirational stories or pictures of people smiling at how great everything is going to be. This book is not that. This book gets real, up-close, and personal. And it engages with you as the unique person you are. Let me hold your hand on this journey. It may be a bumpy ride, but it is well worth it.

It's not going to be yet another diet book, that's for sure. Addiction is about taking control of yourself and over your life. Let me show you how.

Part 1: Mastering Self-Awareness

By becoming self-aware, you gain ownership of reality. In becoming real, you become the master of both inner and outer life. —Deepak Chopra

Chapter 1: Step 1—Remind Yourself You are an Addict

"Wow—that sounds a bit harsh, doesn't it? Isn't that a bit negative? How will that help me?"

Yes, I can hear you thinking all of that. And I agree that building someone up is so much more effective than breaking them down. We will talk about that later. For now, the bottom line is that if you have been struggling with your weight for a long time, with no long term results, you have a problem.

There are two main reasons why weight loss may not happen for you.

The first reason could be you have a physical issue, like an underactive thyroid, Cushing's syndrome, or you are on medication that causes weight gain, and this is something to certainly discuss with your general practitioner if you suspect this. If your meds are for anxiety, depression, and stress, you may overlap and be affected by both reasons.

The other main reason we gain weight and cannot keep it off is that we are eating our feelings. Emotional eating and food addiction often go hand in hand, and no amount of healthy dieting, or exercise, is going to make a difference. Underlying this issue are mental and emotional challenges that desperately need addressing.

So, you need to look yourself in the mirror and recognize the key struggles that are blocking your path to weight loss. The first three steps I will give you are about being self-aware. You won't be able to stick to any action plan for weight loss if you don't admit who you are and face what is going on inside you.

Some of us are emotional eaters, but not food addicts. However, these folk have stuff under control and are generally not overweight. They just eat for pleasure and know when to stop and balance things out. They have other healthy lifestyle choices that offset the occasional lunch at grandma's house, complete with dessert.

For the rest of us, recognizing you are a food addict is the first step. Addictions are not logical. Every addict, including food addicts, know it is unhealthy and risky and we still stay overweight or even obese.

What is an Addict?

In simple terms, it is when you feel compelled to do something to help you feel better. When you are emotionally and mentally driven to perform an act, or series of acts, that help you numb bad feelings, and when those same acts are harmful to you, or those around you.

Addiction is a disease, but it starts in the mind. Even if you are somehow predisposed, or have an addictive personality for whatever reason, the trigger is always thoughts and feelings.

Addiction is a craving. You need a substance or behavior. You obsess about it before and afterward. You cannot control yourself. You cannot stop on your own or without a bunch of help.

Addictions often involve you trying to hide your behavior from others. That bacon sandwich you scoffed at midnight when everyone else was fast asleep, that chocolate bar you eat quickly in the car, or the tidbits you steal off the plates before washing up, are all good examples of this. I have caught myself stealing all the chicken skin off the roast chicken meal before serving it to my family. I mean, what gives? Did I not think they would notice?

Addiction is also a brain dysfunction, based on powerful reward, memory, and motivation neural circuits and feel-good chemicals.

The more you do the thing, the more you need it. The brain desensitizes, and the reward system needs more of the thing to get the same result. You may try to get on top of it, and then you relapse. Think of yo-yo diets as a typical example.

Addicts typically dismiss or ignore the issue. They deny they have an addiction. In a society where being overweight is more the norm, and food is associated with comfort and love, our friends and family may not be helping us to see things clearly either.

However, until people face the facts, often only after serious personal life disruption or loss, nothing can be done. In the meantime, a food addict can sit with permanent health problems: type 2 diabetes, hypertension, high cholesterol, heart attack, stroke, gallbladder disease, sleep apnea, osteoarthritis, breathing problems, depression, and body pain, to name just a few (CDC, n.d.).

If any of this resonates with you, now is the time to stop kidding yourself. You... are... an... addict!

This was a tough realization I had to face about myself. However, only after I faced it and admitted it, could I properly deal with it.

It is time to step up the solutions. But first, let's build some foundational knowledge.

Emotional and Addictive Eating versus Hunger

How do you know the difference?

Well, when you are truly hungry, you will feel specific things on a physical level. These sensations are hard to misinterpret. Your stomach may rumble and feel empty, you get hunger pangs, your energy may feel low, you may be a bit shaky, nauseous, get a headache or battle to focus, and it has been a while since you last ate. The longer you wait to eat, the stronger these signals will get.

When you eat, your blood sugar levels rise, your body gets a boost, and your hunger feelings are alleviated. You may also enjoy the taste and experience of eating. Your body naturally releases dopamine to reward you for the sensible act of fueling it, too. All well and good. That all feels great and should. This is all normal.

Emotional and addictive eating is when you are not generally physically hungry, but you eat anyway. This is not eating as an energy source, to fuel your body only. Food is a source of comfort. You are hooked on the feel-good chemicals released by the brain. The dopamine rush is what you crave. You use food to calm negative feelings when you are tired, stressed, anxious, afraid, or depressed. Or you reward yourself with food as a treat. Sometimes it is also contextual, like a set mealtime, social event, or social spoil. Mom or Gran does love to feed us to show us care and love, doesn't she?

There is nothing wrong with eating nice food and enjoying it. However, when the line blurs between healthy eating and emotionally dysfunctional feeding behavior, we are now in dangerous territory. Overeating, making poor food choices, then starving ourselves, only to binge again, and then attaching bad emotions to it, all puts us firmly into the dysfunctional, addictive category.

Am I Emotionally Eating?

If any of this rings true for you, please at least start considering the possibility that you need some extra help.

1. You eat to feel better.
2. You feel powerless, or out of control when faced with food.
3. You feel shame, or guilt, after a meal.
4. You use food to treat and reward yourself.
5. You eat when you feel stressed, upset, or sad.
6. You eat when you don't feel hungry.
7. You continue to eat after you feel full.
8. You feel stuffed after a meal.
9. Food helps you feel safe or in control.
10. You reach for salty, sweet, or fatty foods in particular.

If you answered yes to any of this, don't panic. Facing the problem is often one of the hardest parts of the healing path.

However, if you have the courage to do so, then the real healing can begin.

Your Addicted Food Brain—How it Works

Before you start beating yourself up about the situation, let's understand a bit about food and our brains.

Food addiction is not something you intentionally fall into. You don't plan to have a problem. But there it is. We need to face it and deal with it.

This is, in part, why.

Our brains have not changed much since caveman days. Honestly, they evolve super slowly. What this means is that they are adapted to a specific food environment. In those days, we had to gather a variety of nuts, seeds, legumes, eggs, insects, grubs, small birds, fish and shellfish, and an array of edible vegetation to get by day to day. It depended on where we lived and what we could find there to eat. Occasionally, the hunters would bring back larger game for us to fill our bellies. Not that often, though. Only later did mankind learn to keep animals and grow crops. Only later did our food source become more reliable. We lived in a food-scarce context originally. So, our brains put in place some powerful motivators and rewards to keep us hunting and gathering and eating, so we would survive.

Those rewards remain as powerful now, even though food is plentiful.

Now, add to the mix our modern food context. There's a lot of it. Many food producers, rather unethically, I feel, don't think so much about our health as their bottom line. So, there are a lot of salty, sweet, and fatty foods available. A lot of 'empty' carbs are high in sugar, but have no real nutritional value, like sodas for example. Fast foods, sweets, cookies, cakes, chips, you name it. They are cheap and plentiful.

These sugars, salts, fats, and highly processed meal options were never meant to be part of our diets. Our brains and bodies don't really know what to do with them. The extreme pleasure and reward of these foods add to our already set food-reward system to make a powerful and potentially addictive combination.

We don't get addicted to bland food so much, do we? Although we may eat it if we are desperate, our first choices are burgers, fries, pizzas, sodas, ice creams, white bread, chocolate, and designer coffees full of sugar and add-ons.

Some scientists at Yale (Becker, 2018), got together and created the Yale Food Addiction Scale. They use neural imaging, which is a real-time image of how our brains respond to various foods. Their results show very clearly that overweight people, in general, have a specific brain reaction to food, in line with the same reaction to an addict taking any other drug of choice. Their results also show food addicts develop a tolerance over time, which means they need more and more of their pleasure foods to get the same feel-good reaction we had when we first ate them.

These really smart researchers have even discovered a genetic mutation in people with eating issues. The brain is trying to reduce the reward function in order to reduce our need for the substance. And what do we do? Well, because all the wrong foods are so easily available, and because we are emotionally dialed into what we eat, we just end up eating more in search of that increasingly elusive reward (Becker, 2018).

Sorry brain—big fail! That poor brain didn't consider our new food environment; the power of advertising; or the availability of cheap, easy, and unhealthy meals. I think we need to hold fast food suppliers more accountable. Even with growing consciousness around this issue, it is still too easy to sell unhealthy food. And bearing in mind that the cost to business and governments in terms of sick days and national health spending, is directly related. I am surprised that many still get away with it.

However, we cannot wait for some sort of worldwide food revolution. We have to step up and take responsibility for our own health.

We need to recognize that our brain and body are not set up to deal with this, and if we don't change, we will get overweight and sick.

We become food addicts.

So, what Now?

Russel Brand in his famous book, *Recovery*, has some lovely exercise questions that are useful to help any addict start building self-awareness.

His step one is to ask, "Are you a bit f*cked?"

Step two is, "Could you not be f*cked?"

Step three is, "Are you, on your own, going to 'unf*ck' yourself?"

What is it that needs to change? What pain, or payoff, are you getting out of not changing? What might it cost you if you don't change? Has this addiction made relationships, work, home life, and daily life unhappy or harder? What have you done in the past to fix this, and has it worked? Step three is about admitting you may need some external support.

There are further steps, but for now, these are the questions you need to get really clear about.

Another important question is, "Are you willing to do what you need to, in order to have this situation healed or changed?"

Do you believe that change is necessary? Do you think it will be easy?

Do you truly get that you do not know how to achieve this, because if you do, you would have done so by now?

If you have seen the results of any addiction in other people's lives, you will start understanding. If you fully and clearly accept that you are a food addict, or could be, and think about it in the same way as any other addict, you need to adopt a similar approach to making a positive change.

For example, what would any doctor or therapist recommend if you were an alcoholic? What would good, informed friends and family suggest?

Would they encourage you, as an alcoholic, to:

1. Stop your treatment just for once to celebrate?
2. Try a 'diet' with light alcohol substitutes?
3. Have alcohol just over the weekend?
4. Just have one drink?

5. Have alcohol only when you are sad, happy, stressed, tired, or angry?
6. Just reduce your quantity intake?
7. Drink all the bottles before you start quitting alcohol?
8. Drink only when you go out and have fun?

I think you know the answer would be a clear and loud, no!

Our Food Environment

The environment does not help. There are plenty of junk food shops around, people surrounding us eating junk food and asking us to join them, and supermarkets with endless choices to eat junk food.

Advertisements push food full of fats, salts, and sugars. They use clever hints, and suggestions, and push you to believe you will be satisfied, happier, and life will be better if you just buy their product. Sometimes, they insinuate that you are not cool, socially connected, or can't be happy, unless you use their product. Who hasn't seen an advertisement with a cool can of soda or beer, chilled and refreshing, or a juicy cheeseburger meltingly deliciously, tempting you? I admit that I want whatever it is they are pushing. I fall for it. If I had that near or in front of me, in the past, I would have eaten or drunk it.

Add to that the fast-food stores on every street corner, the specialty coffee shops with frappes, lattes, and cappuccinos, and the fridges bursting with soda in every corner store.

We also are led to believe that we need to go fully organic, or that fresh, healthy food is expensive. It is if you shop at specialist stores, but you can equally, and easily learn how to shop for basic, healthy stuff, and learn some simple preparation methods that will save money and your life.

We are food addicts literally surrounded by a sea of temptation. So, the journey we need to take is going to need some seriously powerful methods and tools to help you build up your resistance so you can manage your addiction.

Let's face it, if you don't, you could go the way of many other addicts. At the end of the slippery slope of misery is a hospital bed, and then a funeral. I hope you care enough about yourself, and your loved ones, to take this journey with me to turn that around.

Chapter 2: Step 2—Admit You Struggle to Commit to Long Term Goals

Be honest. How many long term goals have you successfully completed in your life?

Some of us have that qualification or built a career. Some of us have lost the weight and kept it off. Some of us have grown happy, stable families. Some of us have mastered amazing skills, knowledge, and abilities.

It is possible.

If you have managed to succeed at any long term stuff, it will definitely help you out now that weight loss is your next big goal. However, if you have yet to achieve big goals, or struggle to reach them, you are among many people who have the same problem.

If you have been struggling with weight loss for quite some time by now, the odds are, you struggle to commit to long term goals as well. Whether or not you have achieved any before, it was probably a matter of extreme effort.

Instead of trying to force the issue, yet again, and maybe failing, it helps to simply accept that this is you. By facing the facts, we can then come up with new strategies, grow our understanding, and put systems in place that actually help us get where we want to be.

Why Do We Struggle?

Part of the problem is how we approach getting what we want in life.

We are primed to expect quick results these days. And, let's face it, weight loss does not happen quickly. Not sustainable weight loss, that is. We also try to do too much at the same time. Food addicts cannot expect to address all the issues at once. It has to be a phased approach. First, we need to get our mental and emotional selves on track, and then the rest can happen. We need to get our food choices right, too, and focus simply on being healthier. Once all that is steadily progressing to our satisfaction, we can start thinking about weight loss and calories. At that stage, having dealt with many of the drivers of our emotional eating, plus feeling physically healthier and stronger, we will be in a more powerful state of mind, and physically more resilient, too.

Instant Gratification

In general, from the moment you decide you want a thing until you get it, it is often a quick process. At the click of a button, and within hours, we can have many items, book trips, learn a new skill, or get a piece of information. If we are hungry, we order online and can get the food delivered in under an hour. Or we stop at the nearest fast-food spot.

Life is fast, fast, fast... People expect service, results, and satisfaction now, not tomorrow or even in an hour. We are all 'on' 24/7, hooked to mobile devices where people can connect to us wherever we are, at any time. When we want to be amused, or informed, or entertained, we pick up our mobile phones and check our social media, emails, messages, and the latest stuff on YouTube or online.

We are not in the habit of waiting. We are in the habit of distraction and quick fixes. This is what we practice every day, for many hours of the day. Both distraction and immediate gratification. When you practice something all the time, what happens? Well, you get really good at it. So, we are good at being all over the place, unfocused, and quickly appeased.

We get used to saying we will do a thing, and then not doing it. Of course, we have all the right reasons and excuses. There is always an excuse that will work for us and get us off the hook with others and ourselves.

Eroded Confidence in Self

The thing is, we are always recording and watching ourselves. Our subconscious mind is a massive recording device, and it does not care about our intentions, dreams, or desires. It records what we think, feel, and do. All the time. If we think or do certain things repeatedly, like giving up on goals, we come to believe that we cannot achieve goals and that the odds of this are very small. We lose faith in ourselves.

We literally teach our subconscious mind to believe that we will not do what we say that we will not, or do not have to, keep our word. We get into the habit of canceling stuff at the last minute, or not doing those things we know are important to our well-being but can always be put off until another time.

We will get around to it, we tell ourselves. I have never, ever found a round tuit by the way. They don't exist.

As a result, you may find you battle to keep your commitments of any kind. Or perhaps you have a series of half-done projects sitting in the closet. Maybe you have become a serial quitter? We are all just too busy to commit to many things. We like to keep our options open. We have become human doings, instead of human beings.

Letting Our Feelings Run the Show

We are also led by our feelings. We don't understand what feelings really are, or how to manage them. They are simply messengers, not our realities. They have something to tell us, but we don't know how to listen, and instead, identify with the feeling and make it who we are, and let it affect what we do. Behind every feeling is a thought, by the way. Thoughts lead to feelings, which lead to actions. However, we will go into this more deeply later.

And so, we allow feelings to rule our lives, instead of being useful tools for us. "I don't feel like making dinner", or "I don't feel like going for a walk now", are words we use when we are looking for reasons not to do a thing. Letting these idle impulses rule us means that we may never do the stuff we need to, because we may never feel like doing it.

Added to the fast pace of our lives, the ease with which we can have many things we want without too much effort, and our whims and impulses, there is another element that holds us back from long term thinking.

We are afraid.

Fear

Fear often underlies our failure to achieve the big, important things in life, like losing and keeping off the weight, writing that book, getting that qualification, or completing any number of things that take extra effort, focus, courage, and tenacity.

We are scared of failing. If we don't ever try, then we don't have to risk failure. We can get by forever saying we will do a thing, but never proving to ourselves or others that, in fact, we can't do it.

We don't want to look foolish.

We don't want to risk failure, so we don't try at all, or self-sabotage ourselves early on by finding excuses.

However, everything needs to be failed at a few times for real learning. We didn't get up and walk perfectly as small toddlers, did we? No, we had to fall down quite a few times first before we found our balance.

Until we accept that perfection is an illusion and that mistakes are a natural part of life, we keep ourselves stuck. If we keep waiting for the perfect time, the perfect feeling, the perfect situation, we will never even start. If we expect perfection, we will always be disappointed.

To progress, we need to find the courage to fall down a bit, accept that it will happen, and keep our focus on what we have gained so far, rather than what we have not yet achieved.

If you never try, you fail anyway. If you do try, there is a chance that positive change will result. It's worth the risk. And everyone will be focusing on their own stuff anyway. Even if you do look a bit foolish, they will soon find a new piece of gossip, and the memory of your mistakes will fade. Odds are, they are too busy making their own mistakes to worry too much about yours.

We are afraid that we will succeed, and that we may have to radically change our lives to do so. We may be losing something in the process, whether it is our sense of safety, a payoff we get for being overweight, or ill (perhaps attention, or concessions), or our sense of self.

We are worried that we will miss out on something better. FOMO (fear of missing out) can stop us from committing to one thing in case something better is out there. Perhaps there's a better diet, exercise regime, or scientific approach to weight loss that if we only just wait, it will pop up and save us.

So, what do we have holding us back so far?

Feelings, instant gratification, food addictions, fear, and self-doubt are hardwired into our subconscious. Oh, and don't forget the endless fad diets and exercise regimes that promise the quick fixes we want, but that long term won't work for most of us.

Wow!

Is there any wonder that we have not managed to achieve our healthy goal weight and stay there?

There are things we need to learn. And they all add up to creating a strong support system to help us meet long term goals. These include learning:

- How our brains and bodies work together. And how one can be used to leverage and support the other in ways you have never considered before.

- How managing our mind is an important tool for our weight-loss goals. Mastering our feelings, knowing what causes them, what to do with them, and how to process, release, and manage them.

- The science behind healthy eating, sustainable weight loss, and how this really works, rather than just calorie and step counting.

- Focus, and not distraction.

- Patience and effort, and not immediate gratification. Understanding what is realistically possible, and how long it might take, and committing to that.

- Getting clear on what is important to you, how to connect this to your long term goals (values) and how to use it to motivate yourself, rather than giving in to your feelings of inertia, fear, or whatever other bad feeling has you in its grip. Using clear, strong rewards to motivate, and robust support systems to help you keep going.

- Resilience, for when we make mistakes.

- Tenacity to help us keep going, no matter what. "You don't set out to build a wall. You don't say, 'I'm going to build the biggest, baddest, greatest wall that's ever been built.' You don't start there. You say, 'I'm going to lay this brick as perfectly as a brick can be laid.' You do that every single day. And soon you have a wall." —Will Smith.

- Courage and insight, so we can face our fears and see that any gains we make are bigger than the risk of failure.

How do we do all of this? I will show you in steps four and five, but for now, it is enough to accept that right now, you may not be able to commit to long term goals. However, soon we will help you strengthen these skills and put tools in place to make it all more likely and easy for you to follow through.

Chapter 3: Step 3—Stop believing you know it all

If what you had done so far had worked, would you not have solved the problem by now? With all you know, and can do, and your skills and abilities, did any of those get you to make a change yet?

No?

Then you need to accept that some serious changes in mind, body, and soul may be needed. Be open to the path I will be taking you on, because I know that this will work for you.

We are all different, and yet there are some generic, foundational concepts that pretty much apply to any food addict. And these are what we are going to get to grips with and start applying in our lives.

I have taken myself from a lifetime of being overweight, obese, yo-yo diets, shame, guilt, and misery into a whole new space of freedom and light.

It took me 30 years of doing a lot of the wrong stuff before I figured it all out. However, for the past five years, I have been able to maintain a healthy weight. It took work, and I had some hard learning curves before I got there. It does not need to be so hard for you.

Myth #1: It's All in the Diet

If you could just find the right one that works for you, then you will be fine. If you can keep your calories below a certain amount, then you will be fine. In essence, this is not untrue. Limiting calorie intake does help with weight loss, but we are learning that diet-based approaches to weight loss are not generally effective on their own.

In fact, diets are often a predictor of eventual weight gain, not loss. Around 85-percent of dieters end up gaining the weight back, and putting on more, within one year (Gunnars, 2019).

This happens for a few reasons.

Firstly, most diets are too restrictive. By approaching a new habit with an "I can't have" mindset, you start off feeling deprived and having to use vast quantities of will-power. This is really hard to maintain for even the strongest-minded people. On busy days, or when you get stressed or tired, it is even harder.

There is a better way to think about your calorie intake, which involves switching the mindset around and putting support systems in place, so you feel less left out and limited.

With many popular diets, even if we get it right and lose some weight, at great effort and energy cost, we simply can't maintain it forever. The diet is not a sustainable lifestyle change or fit. Also, many diet gurus base their diet on a specific approach, for example, banting, ketogenic, raw food, and so on. While the science they base it all on is not wrong, it often is not complete, or it works for certain physiological and mental types and not others. Even people in research studies who do well at first, often put the weight back on, once the study ends and all the intense support, monitoring, and controls fall away (Schmerling, 2020).

Diets can also be bland, or outside of our comfort zone with foods we don't know how to prepare in tasty ways. They also often require large changes to our eating patterns that we try to apply all at once, with no understanding of how to maintain good habits.

We get busy, we get distracted, and we eventually stop trying. And then the weight piles back on. And we start to think that no diet will ever really work. And we are right, in a way.

A large-scale research study into popular diets like Atkins, Weight Watchers, DASH, Jenny Craig, and the Mediterranean diet, tracked dieters over a year. They found that in general, weight, cholesterol, and blood pressure improved around six months on, but by around one year, the results were less impressive. The only diet that had lasting results was the Mediterranean diet, which showed reduced cholesterol past the year mark as a result of following it for a time. Most dieters on all the diets had regained the weight. Not because the diet itself was bad, but because it wasn't enough on its own to get to and maintain a healthy weight (Schmerling, 2020).

It seems to matter less which diet you pick, than whether you are able to maintain it long term. And to do that way more is needed than just will-power, an eating plan, and a recipe book. There are so many factors involved, and all of them need to be addressed. This includes understanding the root beliefs behind self, weight, and food, emotional eating triggers, managing moods, sleep quality, support systems and tools, and more. A holistic approach is needed.

Myth #2: You Can Exercise It Off

We often have an inflated idea of how much exercise influences weight loss. Let's just look at the figures to get some perspective here.

One serving of a classic beef burger with cheese and a small order of fries, one bagel with plain cream cheese, a large Belgian waffle with one-and-a-half tablespoons of maple syrup, a Big Mac, four slices of bacon, a Snickers bar, or a Starbucks Frappuccino with 2-percent milk and whipped cream on top, all come, individually, to around 500 calories. This is just to give you a basic idea of what 500 calories might look like (Lifehack, n.d.).

Okay, now how much exercise would you need to do to burn that off?

You would need to do an hour of vigorous belly dancing, Zumba, or aerobic dance. Or you could try an hour of vigorous swimming, going at a punching bag for about 70 minutes, or riding your bicycle outdoors for about the same amount of time.

Running, for about a 150-pound person, will burn about 13 calories per minute, which is 792 per hour, if they spend that whole hour consistently fast (Uttekar, 2021).

Five-hundred calories are about a quarter of the average person's required daily intake. However, overweight people obviously eat way over their required amount, and are in no shape to do intense, vigorous exercise in any case. If you are already overweight, starting a crazy, loaded exercise plan can be overwhelming. Not to mention, you feel bad in that tight lycra sports gear in front of the judgy eyes of others, and you already aren't that good at sticking to a training schedule. And your body and bones ache; you are tired, and over it.

Exercise as your main plan for sustained weight loss is, again, not the best approach. It would simply take way too many hours to work off the extra calories for someone starting out on a weight loss journey. It is way better used as part of a holistic weight-loss approach.

It is great for mood management, lowering blood pressure, increasing metabolism over time, better sleep, and many other things, but on its own, it won't do the trick. Exercise is more for endurance, muscle strength, and overall health, than for weight loss, to my mind.

Exercise is also a triggering word for many people who struggle with weight. The very word can shut some of us right down in disgust.

Not only do we overestimate how many calories we burn with exercise, but we also tend to eat more when we do, and often get less active in the remainder of our day, because we believe we have exercised enough.

We can eat hundreds of calories in just a few minutes, and that means that whatever we burnt off with exercise, we can quickly pack back on and more.

So, if we want to include it in our lifestyle plans, we need to be smart about it, and link it to health goals that don't just include weight or physical goals, but also mental health goals, too. These include better sleep, increased alertness and focus, and a better overall mood and resilience. We also need to gradually phase exercise in, in a way that we enjoy and can sustain. And we need to understand how exercise works with the mind and body, and what kinds work best for our personal goals.

There are loads of ways to make exercise work for and with your weight-loss plans more effectively. And we will look into all of this in-depth in the "how-to" part of this book.

Myth #3: If You Are Doing It Right, Weight Drops Off Consistently

It would be great if from the moment you decided to start losing weight, it all started melting away. In a way, this is often what we expect, especially when we are used to getting whatever we want very quickly.

Unfortunately, our bodies don't care about our wishes and personal timelines. They took time to put on the weight, and by gosh, they will take their time to lose it.

This is part of getting your mindset right from the beginning. Those fad diets that have you eating two peas and a cube of cheese a day may drop the pounds quickly, but as we know, they are hard to maintain and unhealthy in the long run.

As a rough guideline, the average (read 5 feet 4 inches, and 126 pounds) adult woman needs around 1,600 to 2,400 calories every day to maintain weight and meet energy needs. The average man (read 5 feet 10 inches, and 154 pounds) needs 2,000 to 3,000 calories. To find your own requirements, you can use any one of the online metabolic rate calculators. These factor in height, age, weight, body size, activity level, and your weight loss goal to calculate a recommended calorie intake. If you know your body fat versus lean mass ratios that can help, too, as more muscle burns more fat (Fetters, 2020).

Having this mind and tracking each meal on some sort of weight-loss app, soon shows you where you are going wrong, and what calorie choices to start replacing or avoiding.

In general, to lose weight you need to take in fewer calories than what you require to maintain and meet basic energy expenditure. This will depend on your specific criteria and goals as well.

You may also see fluctuations in the scale, and often these depend on water intake, what time of day it is, and how much food you have just eaten. It's always best to weigh in at the same time of day to get a clearer idea, for these reasons. These small ups and downs are nothing to be worried about in the beginning. My dismay whenever the scale went up a pound or two in a day was demotivating, and in reality, was simply based on incidental stuff anyway. Although I never stopped checking the scale as part of my continued motivation, I had to learn all about this particular myth to keep things in perspective.

We rather look for a consistent trend in weight as an indicator that what you are doing is working, or not.

However, there's more to it than that, of course. Biology is complex, and changeable, as any doctor will tell you.

Weight loss has four phases. First, as you start limiting calories, you enter a calorie deficit. That's if you can stick to your recommended daily intake.

Glycogen (sugars) stored as fats fuel your body. In a calorie deficit, you start burning off fat stores in the liver, and more slowly, any fat stored in muscles.

Water stores also add to overall weight and thus are not to be confused with fat loss. Water is not something you want to reduce when trying to lose weight, by the way.

The next phase is actual fat loss. This is where phase one has found a sweet spot, and if you are maintaining your calorie targets, you start steadily losing weight. Losing between 1 to 2 pounds per week is a good rate to aim for and expect.

At some point, and we can't say exactly when, you will hit a weight loss plateau. Suddenly, despite sticking to your calorie target, and doing all the right stuff, your weight stops moving. It's basically your body waking up and realizing that you are losing weight consistently, which it reads as a possible threat to survival. So, it slows right down and does stuff to stop all this change.

Don't despair. If you stick with what you are doing, eventually your body will realize you are not under threat, and the plateau will end. There are ways to speed this up, like occasionally increasing calorie intake or stepping up exercise (energy expenditure) for a bit.

The last phase is metabolic recovery, where your body finds a new normal. At this point, the scale may go up, but just stick to your new healthy lifestyle. Eventually, it will settle, hopefully somewhere around your goal weight. Once you hit goal weight, you can increase your calorie intake to a non-weight-loss amount, and simply maintain it there, in that way (Lift and Live 2018).

Myth #4: All Calories Are the Same

Although we measure calories using standard numbers, so it can seem that 200 calories of soda are no different from 200 calories of Brussels sprouts, not all calories are the same. The source of your calorie choices makes a big difference to how the body processes that food source. All of this affects how hungry, or full, you feel, and how soon you need to eat again. This, in turn, affects how much you eat in a day, and how hard or easy it is to stick to your calorie intake goals.

A fat calorie is not the same as a protein or carbohydrate calorie.

Simple sugars from refined foods and liquids process quickly through your body and can leave you hungrier than ever, almost right away. These are things like sugary sodas, coffees, sweets, cakes, cookies, alcohol, and so on, which give you that sugar rush, but don't fill you up much. Some fruits, although richer in fiber, also deliver simple sugars faster, like citrus fruits, and melons. These are still better than drinking a sugary soda, but fruit juices need to be monitored for this reason.

Calories from slow-release carbohydrates, whole foods like vegetables and fruits that have a low-calorie density, but added fiber and mass, and proteins, all help to make you feel fuller for longer. Liquids like soups and smoothies based on broth, and vegetables, or fruits like berries and bananas are also great to help you feel fuller for longer.

Also, carbs don't necessarily make you fat. While a low-carb, high protein diet will help lose weight, the whole anti-carb drive has been misleading. Actually, carbs found in whole foods are very healthy. It's the refined carbs and simple sugars that you want to avoid.

And lastly, eating fat does not make you fat. It is calorie-dense, so eating too much of it will be a problem, but if you restrict and monitor it, it can even help you lose weight. The naturally occurring fats in protein-based food are fine, within reason. You need some fats for various body functions. It's the added fats in junk foods that are the problem.

Myth #5: Being Overweight Is All About Willpower

Thinner people tend to look at overweight people and are quite critical, especially if they have not followed their own weight loss journey. It's easy to judge when you have not walked in those shoes.

Those of us who have had to shed many pounds, and keep it off, are a lot kinder about how we judge others, and ourselves. We know that being overweight does not necessarily mean you have no self-control or have no willpower.

In fact, scientists have now found genetic markers that many overweight people have, which decreases the reward they get from food (meaning they need to eat more to get the same feelings of satisfaction), have higher levels of ghrelin (the hunger hormone), and lower levels of (or even resistance to) leptin (the satiety hormone that tells you when you have had enough to eat). There is a fat-mass and obesity gene (FTO) that is now found in around 43-percent of the population (Sicat, 2018). Emotional eating, as we have mentioned before, is a huge problem as well, with many overweight people having unresolved pain or life challenges they are not yet equipped to meet, and who use food to help them feel better.

So basically, you could be one of the unlucky ones whose biology or mind makes weight loss that much harder.

While we can't necessarily test our genetic markers that easily or cheaply, it might pay to get a few physical tests to rule out other possibilities. There are several medical factors, like an underactive thyroid, polycystic ovary syndrome, or even depression and anxiety (and the related medications), that also pack on the pounds.

So no, weight loss (or gain) is about far more than just having a sweet tooth or no will-power. That is why we need a holistic approach to help with physical, mental, and environmental factors altogether.

Myth #6: You Have to Eat Regularly to Lose Weight

Look, the fact is that if you are so self-disciplined that you always eat a good breakfast, the odds are that this same self-discipline would extend into other areas of your life and make weight loss easier on the whole.

However, people who do intermittent fasting would argue that small, regular meals are not needed.

Maintaining blood sugar levels is definitely important, but it comes down to learning your body's cues. Basically, eat when you feel hungry, but don't wait until you are starving hungry, or you will overeat. On a scale of 1 to 5, where 1 is not hungry at all, and 5 is ravenous, you should aim to eat around the 2 or

3 marks. That may mean planning ahead or carrying healthy snacks when you are on the go.

And then when you feel full, or actually a bit before that, stop eating. It takes around 20 minutes for your stomach and digestive system to register that it has had enough food. So, eating slower, or stopping eating after a certain portion size, is a better way than simply eating until you can't eat anymore.

Myth #7: Diet Foods and Supplements Are the Way to Go

Sadly, many processed foods with the word 'diet' on the label are high in additives, salts, and even sugars. Low-fat, gluten-free, and fat-free foods may contain chemicals that are quite bad for you.

'Healthy' foods like high-fiber cereals may contain added sugars, and even health and energy bars may contain a load of unhelpful stuff that creates a chemical storm in your body. Not all marketing is honest, folks.

As time-consuming as it might be, it pays to read your food labels. Added fats, salts, and sugars are a no-go.

Things to look out for are sodium (salt), saturated fat, trans fat, sugar, corn syrup, dextrose, maltodextrin, molasses, glucose, fructose, maltose, sucrose, aspartame, hydrolyzed protein, monosodium glutamate, BHA/BHT, artificial colors, and potassium bromate (American Council on Exercise, n.d.). Ingredients are always listed with the order of amount, with the greatest quantities coming first on the list.

This list is not exhaustive, but in general, it is just better to eat whole foods, prepared fresh, and prepared without added oils and fats. Our bodies get confused when we put a lot of chemical, alien additives into them, and these have a variety of effects that may make weight loss, and health in general, harder.

It does not mean you can never eat out, buy fast food, or a ready-made meal. However, stay conscious of your choices, and keep the added sugars, fats, salts, colorants, and other preservatives and product-enhancing stuff to a minimum.

Then, supplements are massive in the weight-loss industry. They often contain caffeine, vitamins, minerals, fiber (which does fill you up and reduce hunger), and various herbs.

Some suppress appetite, and some have other effects that are based on herbal additives. Many supplements have been put through very limited trials, and often supplements are recalled, because it is later found there are health risks attached. There are a few supplements that may be safe and have a small effect on weight loss, but many require you to add a healthier eating plan anyway (Kubala, 2018).

If you really want to go this route it is best to get proper medical advice first. But honestly, you are more often better off just increasing water, fiber, and eating whole, naturally occurring foods that help you stay fuller for longer.

It can be tempting to go for a quick fix, but as long as you are doing that, you are truly delaying your real weight-loss journey.

Ultimately, combining quality sleep, monitored and healthy nutrition, increased movement, and physical activity levels, and use mood and stress management techniques, you are more likely to lose weight, than if you do any one of these, or ascribe to any of the above myths.

Chapter 4: What's Your Story?

To really understand what is going on for you, as a unique individual, and what your specific food challenges are, we need to dig into your story.

Like with any addiction, there is always a root cause, or even a number of them, that triggers and creates unwanted eating behavior. It's all very well to understand how to eat healthily and get in your exercise and sleep. These are all important supports to weight loss and control. However, if you don't pay attention to the emotional side of things, in my experience, no amount of calorie counting or anything else will work.

Only getting to the root of what is going on in your head and heart will give you the resilience, skills, and fortitude to carry through with the lifestyle changes you want to make.

What Does Food Mean to You?

We all have our own programming around food. What we have been taught to believe, and what we have internalized around food and eating will play a large part in how we interact with it. And that is different for each one of us.

Our root, or core beliefs, start developing from day one of our lives, and are strengthened throughout childhood. They are not universal, and more assumptions based on what we are told and taught, our experiences, and how our primary caregivers themselves see and react to food as well. The problem is, we mistake these assumptions for facts, and often think everyone thinks and feels the same way we do, or that this is just how things are.

These core beliefs entrench themselves within us, and subtly dictate our choices. The good news is, once we realize this, we can expose and analyze them, and leave any unhelpful ones behind.

Studies show that many people with weight problems, also have faulty, unhelpful core beliefs around food (Dingemans, 2009).

To understand a bit more, let's take a look at some common root beliefs people hold around themselves and food.

1. Shame or low self-worth. The core beliefs of, "I'm not good enough. There is something wrong with me. I am ugly. I am unlovable. I don't deserve [x]. I have to be or do something in order to be loveable. I will never be loved", will resonate with you if this is your challenge.

2. Lack of self-control. The core beliefs of, "I can't do this. I can't control myself. I never do what I say I will, or plan to do", fall in this category.

3. Feelings of incompetence. Things like, "I'm stupid. Everyone is better than me. I can't handle life. I can never get this right. I am a failure."

4. Vulnerability. Thoughts like, "Bad things always happen to me. Life is scary."

5. Mistrust. "I am not safe. People will hurt me. People will use me. I can't trust anyone to be on my side or help me."

6. Abandonment. "People always leave me. Loving others hurts. I am so alone."

7. Perfectionism and uncompromising standards. "I have to be the best at all times. I have to be, or at least appear to be, perfect. If I'm not perfect, I'm a failure. If I'm not perfect, I won't be loved."

These underlying beliefs about our worth or existence make it more likely that you will seek solace in food, use it as a means of controlling your world, or playing out our feelings of shame and reinforcing negative core beliefs. For example, "There is something wrong with me", is the core belief that could lead someone to use food to prove this through food addiction or an eating disorder. Remember that if we believe something like any of the above about ourselves, it is not always a conscious thing, and we tend to make choices that support whatever it is we are believing, even if that makes no logical sense, and is potentially destructive to us.

Faulty core beliefs can lead us to turn to food in place of love, to use it to self-soothe, self-destruct, distract, or amuse ourselves.

There are also core beliefs we have about the actual act of eating that further complicate the issue.

1. We equate food and eating with love and connection. A mother feeds her children, a family sits down to connect and eat together, we give chocolates and sweets to those we care about, and we show our love by preparing delicious dishes for our loved ones. Who, in turn, feel compelled to eat what we make to show their care for us in return. Anyone who has ever felt compelled to eat Granny's high-calorie apple pie, or Aunt Lily's three-

chocolate fudge biscuits, will know exactly what I mean here.

Not to mention that in many cultures throughout history, breaking bread together conferred safety and acceptance of a guest in your home. We have all these traditions and core beliefs working against us if we are trying to conquer food addiction.

Rather, encourage your family to turn to activities in place of food, and educate them around healthier choices if you can. A cricket game on the lawn, a charity event, or a walk down to the park together are all just as connecting as sharing food and drink.

And if you can't convince Aunt Lily to stop offering you those biscuits, then you need to get some words ready to head off the food pushers.

2. We equate food with fun, joy, and entertainment. Most social events involve some form of special catering. If you attend the event, you will appear ungracious or unsociable not to eat what has been provided.

   In these instances, learn to only choose the healthier options, and limit your portions. Or keep away from the food table and spend your time with a healthy cup of herbal tea or glass of sparkling water, in your hand, instead.

3. We equate food with healing on a physical and emotional level. A cup of tea to calm your nerves, a piece of cake to cheer you up, or a chicken soup to heal a cold, are commonly accepted as things that make you feel better. Of course, I am big on nutritional healing, and healthy food obviously does give you energy,

strength, and nutrients that your body can use to fight off illness. So yes, healthy food is healing, but not all food fits that category, as we know.

However, the line blurs when we start turning to unhealthy options as a means to feel better. There is no doubt that sweet, salty, and fatty foods trigger our brain reward system, and release extra dopamine, not to mention, taste great. It is easy to then think that this is the way to feel good fast, but in reality, we know our health takes a knock, we put on weight, and our self-esteem and confidence plummet, too.

4. So many of us believe that cleaning your plate means you are mature, responsible and all that good stuff. Only babies and ungrateful, wasteful people leave food behind. This is a faulty core belief, leftover from days when food was scarce and expensive. World War II, economic recessions, and even recent hardship caused by the Covid epidemic may lead families to force this issue. If you are a member of the clean plate club, you are likely eating past the point that you are full. You get used to eating a certain portion size that may be larger than what your body actually needs.

   Rather, only eat when you are hungry, eat slowly, and eat until a few bites before you feel full. As we know, it takes 20 minutes for our stomachs to register fullness.

   If we learn to listen to our bodies and follow their cues, we are setting the stage for a much healthier approach to eating.

5. You have to eat at certain times. While keeping your blood sugar levels fairly constant is a great idea, your body will tell you when you need to eat. You don't have

to do breakfast, lunch, and dinner, on someone else's schedule. Unless your body tells you that you are hungry, don't eat. Maybe, limit the shared, family meal to once a day, or once a week.

Lastly, we tend to think that whatever diet we grew up with is the way to eat. Many people don't stop and question how things have always been done. Once you know what healthy eating is, and is not, it may be time to review it all considering this.

Practical Exercise: What Are My Core Beliefs?

Answer a few of the following questions, to help you uncover unhelpful core beliefs.

1. Make a list of any of the beliefs mentioned in this chapter that you feel resonate with you.
2. Think about your past, as far back as you can remember. Make a list of any critical or traumatic memories, and what these may have made you feel about yourself.
3. What automatic negative thoughts do you have about yourself whenever something goes wrong? List as many as you can think of. If you cannot think of any, watch your thoughts for a few days to see what may come up. Keep a notebook handy, because if you don't write it down right away, the odds are, you will forget.
4. Finish the following sentences:
    a. I am...

b. People are...

c. The world is...

You can come up with multiple answers for each of these leading statements.

5. Next, think about food in general, and finish these sentences:

    a. Fixed mealtimes are...

    b. Food is...

    c. I eat, because...

    d. Fun food is...

    e. Boring food is...

    f. My favorite food is...

    g. I hate eating...

    h. Cleaning my plate at every meal is...

    i. I eat when I feel...

    j. I eat when I go to...

At the end of this exercise, you will have a long list of sentences that will point to possible core beliefs you have about yourself, and about food. Some of these things you may not have been consciously aware of before, or never really gave it much thought.

Now is the time to do so. Now you have uncovered a few root beliefs and you can start taking charge of your choices and life from a more informed place. Look at each core belief and ask yourself:

1. Is this true?
2. How do I know for a fact that this is true?
3. What does this sentence actually mean to me? I am saying this, because...?
4. What would other people say about this? (Consider actually asking a range of people)
5. Is this belief helpful to me? How?
6. What are the advantages of believing this?
7. What are the disadvantages of believing this?
8. Can I reframe or rephrase this belief in a more helpful way? For example, if your belief is, "I never get anything right", can you think of any time when that was not true? Can you rather say, "I am learning to do better"?
9. If the belief is true, but not helpful, what can you change now, today, to start shifting it toward a more positive state?

What Are Your Triggers?

Our core beliefs will influence our choices. That is a fact. And our core beliefs, plus events or situations, equal a trigger that can set off poor food choices and addictive behavior.

Practical Exercise: Eating Triggers

Keep a food diary for a period of about a week.

Each time you eat, note:

1. What you ate.
2. When you ate.
3. Why you ate it? Choose from the following or add your own reason.
    a. You wanted to feel better.
    b. You felt powerless, or out of control.
    c. It was a treat or reward.
    d. You felt tired and wanted a pick-me-up.
    e. You felt stressed, upset, or sad.
    f. You wanted to feel safe or in control.
    g. You were simply hungry, no feelings attached.

At the end of your week, see if you can spot a pattern. For me, I was eating when I felt bored, for the pleasure of the taste, and also to please others in social situations. I also ate when I felt tired, unhappy, or stressed.

These were my most common triggers. Beneath my stress, boredom, and unhappiness, in particular, were other core beliefs I held about myself and the world I lived in. So, knowing what these were, and turning them around, helped immensely with removing the trigger and the desire to eat when I didn't actually need to. By healing and removing the core belief part of the equation, it no longer added up to bad choices.

It helped me identify when my emotions needed attention, and then I learned to use other methods to feel better, rather than reaching for a cheeseburger or cake.

Processing Tricky Feelings

If we agree that many eating triggers are not truly hunger-related, we are left with looking to the mind and heart for answers. Food addiction, like any addiction, is most often a problem because we are trying to numb uncomfortable or even painful thoughts and feelings.

Feelings like boredom, shame, guilt, stress, depression, anxiety, worry, and anger need to be faced and processed, in order to defuse those pesky triggers, too.

As mentioned before, we tend to think that our feelings are end results or things in and of themselves. And we think they are always true and an indication of reality or who we are. We may even identify with them. This is actually unhelpful thinking. Feelings can be a result of so many things: our core beliefs, our hormones and physical state, and our thinking. If we can accept that there is a possibility that whatever we are thinking may not be 100-percent true or helpful to us, we have already made progress.

Just being aware of our thoughts and putting them frequently under a microscope is a great start. Then, being aware of our feelings, and learning to watch for them as messengers, rather than facts, is the next step.

Bad feelings are simply indicators that there is something in our life that needs our attention. To know what that might be, we need to look at our thoughts, context, and physical state for clues.

If you are taking care of the basics physically, then you can rule that out. Hunger, illness, tiredness, dehydration, discomfort, and chemical or hormonal imbalances can all affect our emotions, so check for this stuff first. Sometimes, it is as simple as getting a good night's sleep to improve your tolerance, resilience, and mood.

Good things to check on a physical level include:

1. Are you eating healthily? There are also supplements and good mood foods you can choose to help with mood management. We cover all of this a bit later on in the book.

2. Are you hydrating with healthy liquids, and are you drinking enough?

3. Are you getting at least 20 to 30 minutes of some sort of physical activity or exercise every other day? Exercise vastly improves mood.

4. Are you getting outdoors? Fresh air and sunshine are good for the mind and body. The vitamin D we get from sunlight is important for general health and mood management, too. Plus, studies support the fact that getting outside and anywhere near some sort of natural environment is very good for mental health. Beach, forest, mountain, or just your local park are all great ways to get closer to nature and ground ourselves.

5. Are you getting quality sleep? This is super important for weight loss, as well as managing stress and general

mood. Everything is harder to deal with when you are tired.

6. Is it possible that your hormonal levels, thyroid, or some other physical element is out of balance? It might not hurt to get a check-up to rule this stuff out.

We are complex creatures, and our moods are often influenced by a multitude of small things, rather than one big problem. So, when trying to improve and manage our moods, we need to take a multi-level approach and put many smaller support systems in place that all build toward overall inner peace and happiness.

However, we also need to look at bad feelings that are persistent and consistently there. If we identify that we are stuck with thoughts and feelings we don't want, we need to face them and see what they are telling us. Once we have excluded any obvious physical reasons, we need to look at what's going on in our heads. What do these bad feelings mean? And what can we do about them?

Let's look at them one by one.

Anger

When we feel angry, obviously something has set us off. Sometimes, we find we feel angry a lot of the time, and don't really know why. Or perhaps, the smallest thing triggers us, and we blow our tops, only to feel ashamed and regret what we did or said while in the heat of the moment.

Anger is often a sign that there are other root emotions underlying the angry reaction. Figuring out what these are might help to defuse the anger in the future.

Underneath an angry reaction could be:

1. Frustration. You are not getting something you expected or feel you deserve, or something is not happening in the way you want it to.

   In this case, you could ask for what you need, discuss, or negotiate expectations, and also take responsibility for meeting your own needs. Often, we expect things we have not even communicated to anyone. We just think that somehow, if they cared, they would read our minds and know. But of course, they can't. We have to use our words.

   If you are often driven over the top by circumstances beyond your control, like the traffic, that rude cashier, or your screaming toddler, you need to take a step back and evaluate the situation. What can you do? What can't you do? How can you let go of trying to control the uncontrollable? Practice non-reaction to these kinds of life challenges. Practice not acting on the trigger and try one of the methods below to defuse your strong feelings.

2. Hurt or pain that lies beneath the anger means that you need to address the root cause. How can you forgive, let go, and heal? Use the root or core belief work we did earlier to help you or consider getting the help of a professional.

3. Fear, insecurity, or feeling threatened in some way. For example, a mother who sees her child run into the road

may lash out with anger at the child. Beneath that anger is her fear that he may have been hurt. Better to delay the emotional reaction and deal directly with the problem. Is there some way to deal with this fear, for example, by teaching the child road safety?

4. Feeling overwhelmed lowers your tolerance and resilience. This means you need to look at ways to simplify your life, even if just for a while. What can you drop, defer, or delegate? Can you ask for help? What can you do right now to ease the pressure?

5. Feeling guilty or ashamed about something you have done and lashing out as a result. In this case, you need to get clear this is your issue, and your reactions are unfair and unwarranted. You need to create some space for yourself, away from other people who have nothing to do with your guilt or shame and process these feelings. What can you do better going forward? Or what can you do differently? What lesson have you learned? Do you need to apologize or make amends somehow? Once you have taken the lesson, forgive yourself for not knowing or doing better when you didn't have the ability to do so. Because if you did have the ability, wouldn't you have done better back then?

6. Your sense of rightness, justice, or fairness has been challenged. In this case, what can you do to restore order to your world? Can you avoid this situation in the future, or can you perhaps get help to restore justice? Just make sure that what you believe to be right and just is not harmful to others. Check your thinking before acting.

7. Somebody is crossing or disrespecting your boundaries. In this situation, have you communicated what your

boundaries are? Do you even know? These are different for everyone. However, if something makes you feel uncomfortable or unhappy, and it is a reasonable boundary to have, then you have the right to require those around you to respect your wishes. Often boundaries are linked to your personal values, so are you clear on what is important in your life?

If you have communicated your boundaries, and others still don't try to respect them, then how can you protect your boundaries in the future? Can you avoid the person, avoid the situation, or take a firmer (and always calm) stand? What can you ask, do, or not do, to support yourself in this regard?

Think about the last few times you got really angry. What was really going on?

There are a few ways to defuse anger, no matter what the cause.

1. Check your thinking. What thoughts are underneath the feelings?

2. Use delaying tactics to help you not react immediately when you feel angry. Things like counting and breathing, asking for a time out, walking away, going for a walk (or run), or anything that will put some time and space between you and the triggering situation. Once your body has had time to process the anger, you will be in a better mental space to decide what must be done next.

3. Channel your anger energy into an activity. Exercise, doing household chores, completing that work report you have been putting off, or cleaning out that desk.

> Anything active that will distract you from the anger trigger, and work off the energy in a helpful, rather than harmful way will do.

If you find yourself often angry over all kinds of things, this is a sign that you need to look at your thoughts, and context, and consider how to shift them to something more helpful to you. Anger is not who you are, nor is it a way of life that just needs to be accepted. Ultimately, it is your choice to be angry, and you can choose many other, more constructive ways to manage problems in life than that.

"Speak when you are angry, and you will make the best speech you will ever regret." —Ambrose Bierce

"Anger... it is a paralyzing emotion... you can't get anything done. People sort of think it is an interesting, passionate, and igniting feeling—I don't think it is any of that—it is helpless... it is the absence of control—and I need all of my skills, all of the control, all of my powers... and anger does not provide any of that—I have no use for it whatsoever." —Toni Morrison

Depression

If this is not a brain-chemical imbalance, the odds are there is something you are not facing or avoiding, that needs some airtime. What are you not expressing, or what are you suppressing in your life? The best antidote for depression, after getting your physical health basics right, is to check your negative inner talk, and investigate what you are not expressing. This is often a tough process, but simply sitting quietly with the feeling, allowing it, rather than fighting it, and seeing what comes up, can help.

Sometimes, we also just need some deep rest. Take a few days, if you can, to sleep, rest, and heal. And then again, sometimes, we need to get into action, get moving, doing, and being. Only you will know which of these, or which combination, might be needed. And only you can then do it. Even asking for help often requires that you first do so, as others cannot be expected to always be aware of what is going on inside you.

If your depression is persistent, you may need to seek professional help.

Anxiety and Stress

These are some of the leading mental challenges of our times. Most people will admit to feeling anxious and stressed at some point in their lives. Often, we can get into a habit of feeling anxious, or we can allow stress to go unchecked and become chronic.

This is a complex situation, as are most of the feelings we have listed in this section. While I cannot provide a one-size-fits-all cure, there are a few things to look at to help you reduce stress and anxiety.

1. Look at your inner talk. What do you regularly say to yourself when things get challenging or go wrong? See how you can reframe or challenge these automatic thoughts. Over time, if you persist with watching and reframing unhelpful thinking, it does grow less, and its negative impact is reduced.

2. Look at how you can simplify your life. What can you drop off the to-do list? What can you ask someone else to do? What can you put off until later?

3. Get moving to work those stress chemicals out of your system as soon as the stress feelings start. Even a 10-minute walk will help.

4. Get into water if you can. Even if it is just a bath or shower. It is extremely calming. Getting out in nature is also a good choice to relieve stress.

5. Find other releases for big feelings. Art, dancing, a good shout, or cry where no one can hear you or hitting a punching bag or pillow.

6. Look at what is worrying you. Make a list of those things that are extremely likely to happen and carry a high risk. Next, list high risk, but less likely. Then, low risk, but quite likely to happen, and last, the low-risk and unlikely stuff. Then, make two columns on a piece of paper. Start with the high-risk, highly likely issues, and for each one, write what you could do if that thing happens. What can you put in place now, or do at the time? Who could help? What resources are needed? Not everything will have a clear answer, but there is nothing stopping you from brainstorming with friends and family who care.

Shame and Guilt

Guilt is generally a bad feeling based on something you are currently doing, or not doing. Shame tends to be either about past actions, or about some innate quality you have that you believe is unworthy or bad.

Some self-reflection is always needed.

Do you feel bad about something you are, or something you have done?

If it is about who you are, your identity, or something about you like sexual preference, culture, and so on, then you need to address that openly with people who can help you build self-worth and unpack this unhelpful thinking. After all, if something is part of who you are, it often can't be changed and needs to somehow be accepted. What makes us up as people and is simply a characteristic versus an actual harmful action we choose, is truly not a shameful thing. If it can be changed, should it? Depending on the situation, perhaps the answer might be yes. But again, you need to check your thinking here.

If it is a permanent part of who you are and is not harming you or others, then a way needs to be found to be more accepting of it. By harm, we mean a direct impact on physical well-being or mental health, and not just someone's offended opinions or personal set of values.

If it is temporary and harmful, like being overweight or addicted to a substance, then we still need to be compassionate while we attempt to reduce the harm.

For example, we may feel ashamed about our weight. There are many possible reasons for it having become this bad but shaming yourself about it will only lead to bad feelings that will drive you to eat more. And then you feel more shame, and so we go around in a vicious circle. The only way to stop the emotional and mental harm is to learn a little self-love and compassion and drop the shame. You can still take action to improve your health, but without all the self-hatred or ugly thoughts about it.

By acknowledging it, for example, saying, "Yes I know I am overweight, but I am doing what I can about it”, you bring it into the light, and take away its power over you. You don't need to do this with strangers. Perhaps, just start with yourself, and a few trusted people who can support you.

Often, shame is inflicted on us by others, based on their own value systems that may be limited, and are not in sync with our own. If this is not your value system, this is not your pain to carry. So long as you are not harming anyone, this shame is not helpful to you. Find a tribe that will accept you for who you are. You need to learn how to live with yourself, and perhaps practice some compassion for yourself.

If it is about something you have done, you need to look at forgiveness. You cannot change the past, nor do you want to live there, poisoning yourself in the process. The only way through it is to face what happened, good and bad, and see what lessons can be learned. What can you do differently going forward? Who do you need to apologize to, or make amends to?

Guilt is more about something you have done, and perhaps are still doing. It is a good indicator of an area in your life that you deep down feel you could be doing better in. It may, or may not, be 100-percent correct, but only a good look at the situation will help you know this. What can you improve? What is realistic? How can you start today? Who could help you, or what is needed to support this changed behavior?

Loneliness and Emptiness

It is possible to feel lonely in a room full of people. The relief from these sad feelings comes from finding meaningful connections more than just being around people. Who can you have deeper, or more authentic conversations with? Look for these people, seek them out, and plan to spend time with them, one way or another. Also, go to places where people with similar interests to you are likely to hang out.

A sense of connection does not always have to come by physically connecting with other people. You can connect with yourself and your own thoughts, or you can connect with ideas or other people's experiences, via a book or online. Sometimes, reading about someone who has gone through similar stuff as we have, makes us feel way less lonely just like that. You can also connect with nature, or with a beloved pet. Don't limit yourself to only one kind of connection; try them all.

Empty feelings are telling us we need more meaning or purpose in our lives. Find a cause to champion, or a problem to solve. Sometimes, helping others can give us meaning, or creating something. What is important to you, and how are you bringing this into your life? How can you bring more of it in?

It is tempting to fill empty feelings with food or distract ourselves with treats when we feel bored. That is the quick fix, and that is part of your addiction. Look at addressing the cause. Shift just a little outside of your comfort zone and try something new and challenging. Those feelings will soon alleviate, and the urge to eat will be considerably less.

Whatever the underlying bad feelings are, the point is that you need to deal with them first before you can learn to control your eating habits better. Or at least work at both, alongside each other. If you don't face whatever it is your feelings are trying to tell you, you will continue to turn to food as your numbing agent of choice.

The Way Forward

You may be wondering what any of this has to do with lasting weight loss. Well, it has everything to do with it. As a food addict, until you deal with the underlying emotional pain, you will never get real control over your weight gain.

We can't solve all the challenges in a few short paragraphs, but I hope at least that we have given you more insight than what you had before. If any of these emotional and mental issues are ongoing, and you feel you need help, don't be afraid or ashamed to reach out and get the help you need.

As we mentioned earlier, your feelings are not who you are. They need to be seen as messengers that are there to help you heal and grow. Self-awareness leads to better self-management in the end, and this means you get to better control your food addictions.

The 3+4 Method

We have covered the first three steps.

Step 1—Remind yourself you are an addict.

Step 2—Admit you struggle to commit to long term goals.

Step 3—Stop believing you know it all.

We created some self-awareness about what lies beneath our food addiction, so we can start the change at the root of the problem. Now it is time to fully launch ourselves into the method that will make some real change in your weight-loss journey.

The next four steps are the real deal.

Step 4—Gain extreme discipline.

Step 5—Say No to exceptions.

Step 6—Eat healthily.

Step 7—Set No More and Next goals. Repeat!

These are simple steps to understand, but not that easy to achieve. Trust me.

It's not just all about the 3+4 Method, it is not only about the actions, and it is not just about the diet.

It is about you and your discipline to stick with the steps, and how committed you are to start losing weight today and not quit for a very long time. This sounds like a big task. It is, but you can do it. The next few chapters are going to show you exactly how to get it right.

Part 2: Lose weight once and for all

Most of the problems in life are because of two reasons. We act without thinking, or we keep thinking without acting. — Zig Ziglar

Chapter 5: Step 4—Gain Extreme Discipline

No, we don't mean join the Army or Navy. Although it may sound a bit like that, this is not as rigid as you may think.

When we think about discipline, we often attach a negative connotation to it, when really, all it means is being able to behave in a consistent and controlled way. It does not have to mean deprivation, punishment, or any other unpleasant experience. In fact, done right, discipline is your friend.

Discipline versus Motivation

Motivation is a short-term thing. Sure, it can help you meet your goals. Things that motivate us can be external or internal. External motivators can either be to get a reward or avoid a punishment. The old carrot and stick story. Things like pay bonuses, promotions, winning an award, or even the delicious taste of a double-fudge brownie can all be seen as external motivators.

For weight loss, good external motivators might include feedback from a weight-loss support group or doctor, better-fitting clothes, support from your family or friends, or the sight of your slimming body in the mirror. You could set up your own external rewards, like watching your favorite show after a gym session, or taking a day driving in the country for every 10 pounds you lose. You pick the things that excite you for an external reward.

The thing is, external motivation can be inconsistent and often reduces over time. The thrill of the reward quickly wears off. That bonus is spent, the treat is eaten, or the promotion becomes just part of life. It is not enough on its own to keep things going.

Even internal motivation, which is doing stuff we find rewarding, because it speaks to our values and interests, is not as much of a push as we may need to lose weight. If merely wanting to look better in your clothes, or be healthier, was enough of a motivator, wouldn't it have worked for you already, to keep you on track?

When you are tired, stressed, ill, busy, overwhelmed, or just at the end of a full day, your willpower will be eroded. It makes making the right decisions harder, and it makes slip-ups more likely. You can't depend on willpower alone, as we now know.

We're not saying intrinsic motivation is worthless. Quite the contrary. It definitely helps. However, no matter how good your self-motivation is for now, at some point, it will wear off or get tested, unless it is converted into self-discipline.

Discipline, specifically self-discipline, is one step up from motivation. It's long term, and if you can combine internal motivation together with self-discipline, you are set for success.

To achieve this desired state is not just relying on willpower or motivation. Research shows that those who show a strong level of self-discipline, also have learned how to set good habits, and put routines in place. They manage to rise above being ruled by feelings, and temporary setbacks, and keep on going firmly on their path.

"The successful person has the habit of doing the things failures don't like to do. They don't like doing them either necessarily. But their disliking is subordinated to the strength of their purpose." —E.M. Gray

An Extreme Disciplined Mindset

"I could only achieve success in my life through self-discipline, and I applied it until my wish and my will became one." —Nikola Tesla

But how do we get there?

Not in the way you might think. You might have been told that self-discipline is sheer willpower. That if you are strong, and motivated, and have a strong sense of purpose, these things are enough to win through. Those who don't make it either didn't really want to, were weak, or were simply failures.

If we look at highly disciplined people, we see models of perfection. Those guys who wake up every morning and run a marathon, relish their minuscule bowl of granola—all before they get dressed for work. And they seem to enjoy it, too.

Can we even relate to this? Mostly, no. This is because most people only show you the end result, and not how they got there.

The rest of us just look on in disbelief and consider that perhaps there are indeed aliens among us. We have pictures of monks in scratchy sackcloth with whips, stick-thin gurus in loincloths on windy mountaintops, and muscled bodybuilders, ironman style, stuck in our heads.

However, discipline does not actually work like that. It is not will-power + force + superpowers + innate moral character + deprivation + suffering.

I would like you to suspend your disbelief for a little while, and consider my formula to how real, sustainable, and extreme discipline actually works.

Extreme self-discipline = self-awareness + self-compassion and care + support systems + payoffs and benefits + purpose + habits.

Discipline does not have to be painful. To onlookers, it may look like you are putting in gigantic effort and energy, but in reality, after a while of doing what I'm about to teach you, it will feel okay. Perhaps even quite good.

Self-Awareness

Being aware of your thoughts and feelings, allowing them, observing them, and then processing those suckers is key to healing food addiction.

We can get into certain unhelpful habits with our thoughts, or replay negative inner talk, and this can be majorly self-sabotaging.

Our thoughts are the result of all our learning and experiences up until now. However, what we often don't realize is that just because we are having a thought, does not mean it is a true thought. Or perhaps, it is just one of many possible truths. Thoughts could be faulty, have a basis in shaky logic, or missing and unconfirmed information.

We often aren't even fully conscious of what we are actually thinking. And then as a result of all of this, we trigger feelings that may not be that comfortable. We then identify with those feelings, act, and react based upon them, and take them as facts, rather than signs of underlying thought patterns and life situations that need attention.

Only by taking the time to examine our thinking can we develop the awareness of ourselves that we need to start making positive shifts. Only in this way can we start healing ourselves, and thus removing one of the biggest drivers of food addiction.

Practical Exercise: Thought Watching

Get yourself your smartphone, tablet, or a notebook and pencil, and carry it everywhere with you for about a week.

Every time something goes wrong, what thoughts immediately pop into your head about yourself. Note what happened and what these thoughts were.

Also take some time to recall all the negative stuff people have told you about yourself, or that you know you habitually think about yourself.

Lastly, watch out for thoughts you have about the world, the things you do, and other people.

When you have watched your thoughts for a couple of days, you will probably see a pattern emerging and some common themes.

For each idea or pattern, ask yourself if this is true, and how you know that it is. Is there any evidence you can find that counters the original thought? Can you reframe or rephrase the thought, so it is more helpful and less destructive?

For example, perhaps you think:

1. "I am so stupid." This can be reframed to, "I am learning every day, or I have succeeded today at x, y, and z."
2. "I can't do it." This can be reframed to, "I will keep trying, or I will do what I can (even if it is a small amount)."
3. "People are dangerous." This can be turned around to, "Some people are potentially harmful, but many are helpful." Think of some times when you have experienced that help.

There are many sorts of negative things we can become used to thinking. The more we watch for them, and the more we can turn them around, the less they will occur over time. In this way, we also reduce the bad feelings that can come as a result of these thoughts. And lastly, without the bad feelings being triggered, we feel less of a need to numb them with food.

Self-Compassion

With food addiction, just like any other addiction, there is often shame or fear mixed with darker emotions, unresolved issues, and all kinds of moralistic and judgmental thought processes.

We tend to think, because we give into our addictions, we are horrible people, and we can't change.

Instead, we need to take the judgment out of this. By accepting that all of us are fallible, that we make mistakes, give in to our urges, or lack self-control from time to time means that we are simply quite normal.

Acceptance of this, rather than casting blame and shame, is what will help us look at it all more clearly, with a little kindness for ourselves.

A good example of this is that small child (let's say two and under, for perspective) in the checkout queue who is faced, on eye-level, with a range of sweets and chocolates. When they cry, scream, and kick, because Mom takes away the sweet and puts it back, we may not like the commotion, but we do understand that the small child has not learned to behave differently yet.

Yet!

We definitely don't think that child is a permanent write-off. We just know it has some way to go to behave differently. And that supermarkets are right pains for putting the sweets exactly where anyone hungry and waiting will see them.

We can't just use will-power to force our way through not eating. Those of us who have tried this know it just does not work. And then when it does not, we attach the words 'failure,' 'wrong,' 'bad,' and so on. Then we feel worse, and we need to numb that pain, so we turn to our addiction. And write ourselves off in the process.

Just like the small child in the queue, we need help, distraction, support, or method to get us past the candy without the meltdown.

Support Systems

Food addicts need to recognize that if they could do it on their own, they would have already done so. You need to put everything you can in place to help you maintain the discipline you require to win.

Self-discipline does not have to mean you do it all by yourself. You can ask for help. You can use both external support in the form of mentors and support groups, and you can put systems in place that remove the temptations or limit them.

By creating a multi-layered approach, you stand a much better chance of conquering this problem. So, never think that you have to somehow find the willpower of a superhero overnight. You most certainly do not. In fact, the clever and wise person knows when to ask for help to achieve their goals.

Peer support groups can be found in most places, and if you can't find one, consider creating and hosting one yourself. If face-to-face support is a problem, you can also find many great support groups on social media. Join them, mute any trolls (because they are everywhere, even in well-run groups), and use peer support to springboard your motivation, analyze triggers, and inspire you with ideas, meal plans, and so on.

Creating systems for your daily life, like menu plans and shopping so you only have the healthy stuff ready to eat and carrying healthy snacks when you are on the go, all help prevent starvation and binge eating. If you do end up grabbing an extra snack or meal, the odds are that if you only have good choices at hand, your snack is less likely to upset your progress that much.

Another great support to maintain discipline is having a list of distractions ready for those times when you feel extra tempted. Some of mine include:

1. Drinking a glass of water and waiting half an hour.
2. Taking the dog for a walk.
3. Finishing a household chore before allowing a snack.
4. Calling a colleague, friend, or family member for a catch-up chat.
5. Journaling.
6. Meditation.
7. Taking a nap.
8. Scrolling through social media, watching YouTube or anything that will temporarily distract me.

All of these go-to actions are things I keep in my arsenal. When the craving hits, I use one of these first, before I go grab an extra plate of something out of the kitchen.

It also helps to fall back on the mindful question of, "Am I really hungry right now?" If after some time of distraction, you still feel you need to eat, or you notice the obvious hunger cues like a growling belly, nausea, feeling empty, and so on, then don't hesitate to grab that healthy bite. When you are truly hungry, forcing yourself to wait will only make you feel worse, ill, and more likely to binge eat to calm the hunger pangs. So, building a real awareness of your hunger, and keeping it below the level that the hunger monster takes control of, should be part of a good support system.

Choosing a particular friend or trusted person as an eating mentor is another great support. When you feel you are slipping, this might be the person to call. I have also heard of situations where to add extra motivation, the dieter handed over a cash check for a large sum (for example $2,000) with the agreement that the mentor could cash it in if they slipped up in their food management goals. That may seem a bit extreme, but it is a good incentive to not give in to temptations.

Purpose

Staying clear on your goals is a large part of a disciplined mindset.

We only do that which is important to us. So first we need to get clear on what this is. What are our values, and why do we want to be healthier?

Check in with yourself. Are your goals truly inspiring and motivating for you? On a scale of 1 to 10, where does the goal sit? If it sits below a 7, consider if there is another way to look at this that can make it feel more urgent for you. For example, "I want to be healthy for my family" can be rephrased as, "I want to be active enough to play ball with my son, and to be healthy enough to be alive to see my grandchildren one day."

Practical Exercise: Finding my Weight Control Purpose

Your values will be specific to you. But it may seem a little confusing at first. How do you get clarity?

Take a look at this list of weight-related values and see if anything resonates for you, and also check in to see how much it inspires you.

1. To look good. To be able to buy off the rack, or to know your clothing size, and to also feel okay with what that size is. To be happy with what you see in the mirror, naked or clothed. Perhaps to attract the interest of others by achieving a more attractive and pleasing shape and size. This value can be both personal to you in that you wish to look good to yourself based on what you believe to be acceptable, and also based on common social norms of what society has decided is visually appealing, or sexy and attractive. These norms have varied widely over the ages, so they aren't an absolute standard. Around a century ago, and more, having some extra curves was seen as very appealing, and to this day this is so in many cultures.

   However, we might want to feel sexier and more attractive in the time and place where we find ourselves. We aren't fat-shaming or arguing the point around what is or is not attractive here. We are simply pointing out that having a certain look might be important for you. If that is so, own it as one of your goals.

2. To feel good. To have inner calm and peace, and to not be led by faulty thinking and destructive emotions and triggers. To not have to rely on anything to temporarily numb bad feelings, but to have the power to help yourself feel better when you need to.

3. To be more active and mobile. To be able to do things with friends and family that currently you are unable to do.

4. To live a longer life. To be there for friends and family. Or simply to enjoy more, rather than have it all cut short by ill health.

5. To fit in and be accepted. To not be or feel judged all the time, because of your weight.

6. To have more energy and feel physically stronger.

I don't know which of these speaks to you but take it and make it your own. Attach positive feelings to the end goal. Visualize what it will be and feel like when you achieve what you want and get very clear on exactly what and why you want to achieve it.

Creating a vision board of your health goals is one way to stay focused and mindful. Or perhaps write up a list of your reasons in the front of a journal, as a screensaver on your devices, or stuck on the fridge and bathroom wall.

Habits

Much like with willpower and motivation, we think that setting habits are a simple matter of just pushing through until it comes right. Sadly, this limited approach also means that most of us battle to get rid of those bad habits we don't want or create good ones for ourselves.

Our brain is a funny thing. The more we think about or do a thing, the stronger the neural connections become. Like a path walked over a field, we find it easier to walk the well-trodden way, free of obstructions, clear and easy, rather than forge a new one. This is why certain things are easier to remember, or we do them automatically, because they have been repeated enough that the neural path is strong and clear. Our brain can access this stored information quickly and easily. With concepts and ideas, we talk about types of memory. When it comes to actions, we talk about habits.

We need to apply our understanding of the brain, and how habits are formed, in order to know what we need to do to create the weight-loss habits we need, to support our new disciplined approach.

First of all, we cannot just stop a habit. That takes some kind of godlike power not many of us have. What we can do is replace a habit. That means, if your habit is to start the morning with a coffee full of sugar, you could replace that with plain coffee with low-fat milk.

It is also hard to replace a habit with something less rewarding than the original habit. This means, you could consider replacing that coffee with herbal tea, but it would have to be a darn tasty one with its own caffeine kick. Think green tea with berries, or chai spices perhaps?

Another clever habit creation or replacement trick is habit bundling. This means, taking an existing habit and adding another action to it—one that you also want to habituate. Often, if you take a thing you don't want to do so much and bundle it in with something you already do (and enjoy), it makes it easier to habituate the new thing. For example, perhaps I love my morning coffee and have it every day. That's an existing habit, right? I decide to bundle a new behavior and add a daily weigh-in while I wait for the kettle to boil. Very soon, the new action becomes automatic, too, and I don't even think twice about climbing on that scale right before my coffee.

The next thing to know is that habits do not take a set time to become automatic. There's a story of 21 days for a habit to set, which was based on the findings of a cosmetic surgeon who noticed it took around that time for his patients to get used to their new faces. He extrapolated that to all new ideas and actions, which was flawed science, to be honest.

It depends on two things. Firstly, how powerful the reward is, and secondly, how consistent you can be in the beginning.

So, for example, say you start smoking during your tea breaks when you stand around with all your smoker work friends outdoors. First, the physical rush and relaxation a smoker gets is a super powerful reward, if not that healthy. Second, the odds of it being consistent are high, as the friends will probably encourage you to join them, even if you hadn't at first intended to.

Let's look at triggers and rewards. The trigger is the thing that comes right before the habituated action. In our example, the trigger would be both the work break, and the friends gathering for a social chat outside. The reward is the body's response to nicotine.

Think about some of your habits. What are the triggers and rewards? Write these down.

Now, think about what habits you wish to replace, and which you could use to bundle other new habits with.

Prioritize which ones get attention first. One new habit at a time is all your brain can realistically deal with. Try to change too much all at once, and you know that it becomes super easy to give up on the lot the minute you slip with some of it. So, set one habit at a time. Only once you find yourself doing that thing automatically, without having to think about it, you are then ready to start on the next thing.

Yup, we didn't say this would be quick. However, slow, and steady wins the weight management race.

Consider how you might like to manipulate the trigger for brand new habits. For example, if whenever you go past Starbucks, you just have to stop and get a sugar-filled latte, then you can realistically say seeing Starbuck is your trigger.

You could then choose to take another route, cleverly removing the trigger, and even consider replacing the sugary option with a healthier one.

Next, think about what the habit's reward will be. Studies show that physically based rewards are the most powerful and quickest to set a habit. Think sensory pleasure. That could be tasting, seeing, touching, smelling, or even hearing something you really like. It could also be taking a nap, meditating (for those of us who are hooked), watching an episode of your current favorite series, playing with your pet, or just standing outside in the sunshine for a few minutes.

Take a moment to list all the sensory and physical pleasures that you could use as rewards for your new weight-loss habits.

Make a list of your new, desired habits, in order of priority, together with the triggers and rewards.

Before you start out with re-engineering the new you, keep in mind that we need to go for consistency as much as possible. This means, mostly doing new things. It also means letting go of all-or-nothing thinking. If you do slip up, you need to keep going and not give up in a state of self-disgust and negative inner talk about being a failure. Weight loss, and conquering food addiction in particular, can be a lot about just beginning again for as many times as it takes for the new behaviors to stick.

The things that help with consistency are watching that negative inner voice (self-compassion), plus making your new habit extremely manageable, at least at first. For new habits, a morning time slot is best. That is when our decision fatigue is low, and our tolerance and energy is higher. Also, starting out with the smallest time period or simplest option at first makes it less likely that in those first few weeks you will find excuses not to do the new thing. Think patterns of behavior—we want to use the same trigger, same reward, and keep the new habit as simple as we can in the beginning.

So, when thinking about what the new habit may be, pick a benchmark or goal that you find very easy to do, and feel minimal inner resistance to it. For example, the new habit I choose to start with is drinking water before every meal. My trigger will be a phone alarm half an hour before my mealtime, or when I start feeling those first hunger pangs. I will probably settle on the second choice of letting my body lead my mealtimes, as I don't like set meal times too much. So mild hunger is my trigger.

I will at that point drink my water. My reward, of course, will be the meal I have after first drinking that water. Hopefully, I can make mindful choices there, too.

I carry on with this for a few weeks, and before I know it, I am reaching for that glass without thinking about it. Now, I know I am ready to perhaps fill the glass with a bit more water, steadily increasing it over time, as I go.

Eventually, in this way, a new habit is set. And also, quite a useful one for weight management, as that water is not only super important for general health, but also fills me up and makes me less hungry when I eat my actual meal. If I can add listening to my body's hunger cues, and stop eating when I feel full, I will have made a huge step toward good weight control.

Creating new, healthier habits is a slow and steady process. If you use what you have learned here to support that, you will find it a lot easier. And the more helpful, healthy choices we can habituate, the better it will support us in our journey.

If you are able to use your newfound habit-setting skills wisely, and relentlessly, a disciplined approach to weight management will follow. It has to.

It's not just about understanding habits, though. It's also about patience and your mindset. It's about sticking with it, even when you aren't seeing the progress you wanted or expected. It's about developing the tenacity of a bulldog, and the mindset of a mule. If Winston Churchill had given up at any point in WWII, we would be facing a different reality now.

And when they made mistakes, they had contingency and backup plans to help them recover faster.

We need to think about our food addiction in almost the same way. This is a war we are fighting, for our health, our families, and for our lives. We cannot afford to let anything stop us. We need to keep going, no matter what.

Recovery Plans

A truly disciplined mindset is one that accepts that we are fallible. It is one that knows we need to have some self-compassion, and that we need to work on self-awareness as well. To be disciplined, you cannot rely on sheer force of will. You need to put things in place that will support the new choices you wish to make.

Although we want you to work on your self-discipline and have a zero-tolerance approach, we also understand that to err is human. You have to have a backup plan, just in case.

So, what do you do if you mess up?

First, acknowledge it and face it. Name the thing you did. Perhaps even say it out loud.

Then, take the shame and bad feelings out of it. Apply self-compassion and the forgiveness process. Remember, those bad feelings might trigger more emotional eating, so we need to lessen these quickly and as much as we can.

Get some perspective. What was the slip-up? With most eating issues a slip-up is still fixable.

Make amends to yourself. Decide what it is you need to do to achieve that. Perhaps because you ate that doughnut you need to do an extra hour of exercise today, or you will decide to limit a certain food for the rest of the week. You decide what is reasonable, and then make sure you follow through on that. It is so incredibly important to get in the habit of keeping your word to yourself as much as you possibly can.

Plan to limit the slip from happening again. How can you avoid, reduce, or remove the problem? Is there an emotional trigger that needs some more work? Can you ask your boss to buy healthier treats for the break room? What is it that needs to change?

Once you have decided on all of the above, take a little break and go focus your mind on something positive, upbeat, and happy. Remember, we want to reduce bad feelings and not dwell in a pit of gloom and shame.

Practical Exercise: My Recovery Plan

Take some time to write down the possible options. In the left-hand column, list the kinds of slips you have made in the past. Next, list ways you can avoid the issue before you even slip up. Then, in the next column, write down ways you can make reasonable amends for the slip if it were to happen.

And there you have a solid backup plan for yourself. By doing this upfront, it makes you more mindful, and also less likely to turn one slip into a complete fall from grace.

It's time to get smarter in how you deal with your food addiction. You need to have every tool and trick at your fingertips, ready to use as needed. Especially in the early stages, when you are still building self-awareness, healing triggers, setting up new habits, and so forth.

"If you always do what you've always done, you always get what you've always gotten." —Jessie Potter (Woman to Woman Conference, 1981)

Chapter 6: Step 5—Say No to Exceptions

Remember that you are an addict. As we mentioned before, if you think of yourself as an alcoholic, how serious would it be for you to just have a glass of vodka to celebrate?

It would be pretty serious, right?

We all know that in Alcoholics Anonymous they literally have badges and awards for the number of days you have managed to stay 'dry.' That means no exceptions. Not one drink, not even one small sip, or the taste of it in a dessert. For those people who have made drinking into a coping habit, all it takes is one small slip and they could very well turn that slip into a slippery slope back to ruin.

It's a bit of a contradiction, but alcoholics know they need to have a "no exceptions" mindset, as well as having a plan in case they do slip up, because the odds are too high that one drink becomes many. They have to become resilient and keep going, no matter what.

There is no difference as far as food addiction goes. While that one doughnut won't turn you into a drunken, mindless mess, as alcohol can, it still feeds into the whole cycle of using food as comfort, shame, and emotional numbing. That one doughnut, for you, is as serious a risk as one drink to an alcoholic. Especially in the early stages, when you are still doing the personal growth and healing work you need to remove the source of the addictions. That is, until and unless this is on a firmer level, and you no longer feel an emotional need to eat, plus you have your systems and support in place (including what to do to recover from a slip up). Choosing an unhealthy or junk food option "just once" is a very risky and self-sabotaging action.

Even once you have reached your weight-management goals, this is not a sign that you can let go of your self-discipline and control. You may look gorgeous or feel great. However, what about that other stuff I mentioned before? Should you make an exception and eat that piece of cake? Just once? Are you ready to let go of self-discipline and all the progress you have made?

Nope.

You never, and read this carefully, you will never gain back and keep a healthy weight if you start making exceptions in your diet and eat junk food. Even one exception may make you lose control. And that's because you are fighting an addiction.

I did not say this was going to be easy. There will be endless reasons throughout the day to stop your diet and eat junk food. There will be a lot of people surrounding you, tempting you to share junk food with them.

That is why gaining extreme discipline is such a huge part of the 3+4 Method, and why we mentioned it before this chapter. You won't be able to avoid junk food altogether if you are not disciplined. Making a strong habit of making no exceptions is a very important step.

Boundaries

A big part of making no exceptions is learning how to say no, both to yourself and to others. We know that junk food surrounds us. We know that we will be tested at every turn.

We will be tempted in the office break room, at family gatherings, social events, restaurants, movie nights, holidays, and even when we get a bit stressed out or bored.

Getting clear on your boundaries is very important in this food addiction journey because other people may not understand what you are doing or why. They won't get that food is an addiction for you, and they will put temptations in your path without a second thought, with caring and love. This is even harder with food than something obvious like drugs or alcohol, because very few people would think it is okay to offer a recovering alcoholic a drink, or a recovering drug addict a tablet. We have socially become more mindful of this stuff in the last few decades. However, food is such a mixed bag. We need it to live, and we can never do without it. We also commonly use it for social bonding and the showing of love and care. For someone who is not a food addict or emotional eater, this is all fine. However, for those of us who struggle, we need to learn to set food boundaries and communicate them in ways others will understand and respect if we are to succeed.

Boundaries are simply our personal space. It is what is okay, or not okay, for us, specifically. These vary as each person is unique and has a different set of needs and desires when it comes to what they will allow in their lives.

Creating your boundaries helps you get clarity on what you can or can't do, or will, and won't allow. This is especially important when you think about it in the context of your food addiction. As you know, a crossed boundary could mean a slip-up, and that can spell danger and risk to your health goals.

By having these boundaries decided upfront, you are never placed in a position where you are required to make hard decisions on the spot. If you are tired, stressed, or feel put on the spot, at that moment, you may give in to eating or drinking something that is not part of your plan. However, if you have your boundaries already decided, the ability to say no, or make another choice is far easier. This has a lot to do with clarity, external pressures, and also with decision fatigue.

It helps conserve your energy to know in advance what you will or won't do. Then, you don't have to think that hard about it at the time.

You have a right to say no to anything that does not serve your highest good and your new healthy living goals. Having food boundaries is an essential part of self-care. And the boundaries set limits for yourself and others that make life easier for everyone, and less stressful. Once people know what to expect, they can show their respect and care for you by respecting your food boundaries.

A great example is a good friend of mine who is gluten intolerant. I have a stack of recipes for these meals, and when we plan a social gathering where she is invited, I enjoy creating a few gluten-free dishes for her. At the event, I let her know which ones are safe for her, and also let others know, too, so anyone else who wants to eat gluten-free can do so. She feels valued and important, and I get to have my good friend at my home more often, because she feels safe to eat there, and knows there will always be something for her to eat as well.

Practical Exercise: What are Your Food Boundaries?

You will probably need to do some more reading up, especially in the next chapter, to help you with this one. Creating food boundaries will have a lot to do with healthy eating. It can also deal with emotional triggers, and managing your feelings, too.

Answer the following questions:

1. What foods are now on my no-go list? Write these down. Be specific about it.

2. When will I eat, and when will I stop eating? Do I want specific mealtimes or intervals between meals?

3. What portion sizes will I be okay with? And how much of what kinds of foods will I allow?

4. How will I engage with food in a social setting, if another person wants to serve me, or at home when I am relaxing?

5. What situations trigger my eating? How can I avoid these?

6. What contexts make me feel bad about myself. Perhaps, it is best to get off social media, see less of certain friends who won't quit talking about diets and stop looking at all the super skinny models in glossy magazines. List these as part of your food boundaries, too.

7. What are my reasons for all of the above? Get clear on this, in case you ever need to explain or communicate a boundary, because you will have to do so for sure, even if this is just explaining it to yourself.

The next step, once you are clear on all of this, is to get ready to communicate these boundaries. If no one knows what they are, how can they respect them? It may feel rude or awkward speaking up for yourself, but if you don't, who will? Only you know your values and boundaries, and only you understand how important it is to stick to your health goals.

One way of thinking about food boundaries is as if they are 'allergies,' even if technically they are not. You know certain food choices are bad for you anyway, right? If you quietly explain to the host, or caterer, in advance (at least a few days ahead for catering purposes), most people won't ask why, but they will try to meet your needs.

Ways to communicate your food boundaries could include saying:

1. I have to be careful about my health. I can eat [x], but I can't eat [x].

2. I have some food intolerances that make me quite ill if I don't follow them. Will you be able to provide [x] on the day, or can I bring something for myself if that's easier for you?

3. I simply can't eat [x]. (No reasons given).

4. Thank you for offering to dish up my food, but I prefer to do that for myself.

5. I really don’t like talking about diets (or weight), let's talk about [x] instead.

I am sure you can think of lots of other things you could say. You can make a joke out of it and say your doctor, partner or kid will have your hide if you don't do what you need to, or that the price you pay later is just not worth it. Any of these may be true, in any case.

You don't have to give a reason. If asked, you could just say, "I'd rather not go into the gory details”, or "It's such a long story. Just trust me on this one."

We often feel we have to give a reason but saying no truly does not require any reasons. As you grow in self-worth and personal power and freedom, saying no without any explanations gets easier. Of course, if you wish to explain, you can do so. That is the point of being free to share the level of information that is appropriate for you, rather than feeling pressured to explain to others, because of their demands.

I shared my food struggles and new boundaries with a few close friends and my family, and these people served as extra support, especially in social settings. When a pushy person tried to egg me on and persuade me to eat or drink something on my "not okay" list, these support buddies stepped in quickly to come to my defense. They added their noes to mine, and in the face of that, even the most persistent person generally will back off.

Unfortunately, some people don't have much empathy, or are so set in their own ideas that they can't conceive that other people could think differently. Others are just plain bullies who want everyone to fit in and do what they say. Try to avoid these types in settings where food is involved.

Practice saying your 'no's' out loud, in front of a mirror, until you feel more confident saying them. No one is going to reject or abandon you, because you won't (or can't) drink their Christmas eggnog. Most people are not going to make a huge deal and conflict out of you not eating their cake or burgers. If you let people know up front, and in advance, what your food needs are, most people will go out of their way to do the right thing and give you what you need.

However, if someone insists and places that plate or glass in front of you, there is no shame in simply ignoring it. I have even gone so far as to rehome the item far from me, discreetly, to get up and change seats, or to hand it to someone who might want it instead.

Saying no, or simply not eating or drinking what is given, is your right. At first, you may feel a little embarrassed or awkward. However, over time, that feeling passes. There are plenty of other ways to connect to people or show them that you care about them, without eating the same food as them.

We may feel that this is particularly hard, because eating the food that is given to you has been drummed into you as a child. Often, adults even punish children who don't want to eat what is offered, and this can leave us with problems saying no as an adult. Perhaps we are quiet, sensitive souls who are scared of any kind of conflict, or we have not tried saying no very much before. Perhaps we are scared that people will reject us or laugh at us. Recognize it if this is a core challenge for you, and work on facing your fear, and saying no anyway. If it is really hard, start with a few small 'no's' and build up toward the bigger ones. Your confidence and strength will grow with time and practice, I promise.

You are not responsible for other people's reactions, or feelings, in this regard. They are free to make their food choices, as you are free to make your own.

When we don't set, communicate, and defend our boundaries, we may end up feeling resentful, angry, invalidated, violated, and frustrated. And these bad feelings could trigger emotional eating, so taking some time to clarify and share your needs is always a good idea.

Saying No to Yourself

Boundary setting with yourself, or anyone else, can't happen unless you believe that you are worthy of setting them in the first place.

So, figuring out your values and what is important to you is a key part of being able to say no on any level. That, and staying present to why these things are important. If that means putting up pictures of your children on the fridge to remind yourself about why you need to be healthy, or a picture of a fatty liver on your grocery cupboard door for a while to remind you about what your health choices are doing to your body, then do that.

Visual reminders are very effective ways to keep your goals front and center in your mind.

Planning ahead helps support you in this. So does creating and shopping according to meal plans, checking restaurant menus ahead of time, carrying your own lunchbox or snack pack for busy days, and even taking your own dishes to get-togethers.

Saying no to yourself starts with many of the skills mentioned in the previous chapter, on self-discipline. Setting good habits, knowing your reasons, and putting support systems in place for those weaker moments will all help you stick to your goals.

If you feel you might be about to slip up, consider trying one of the following instead.

1. Take a moment to step away and use the mental tools I have given you to calm down, destress, and get perspective.

2. Simplify your food choices.

3. Remind yourself about your health priorities.

4. Remove yourself from the trigger and the food. Go do something else.

5. Remind yourself that this is your free choice for a better life, and why you have made this choice.

Common Food Boundary Violations

These are times when you and your rights are actually being abused, when a bully or insensitive person is violating your boundaries. It may even be someone with good intentions who cares about you but doesn't understand what you are going through.

Here are some examples.

1. Comments made about your weight.

2. Comments made about your food choices.

3. Comments made about your health or the truth behind anything you have said to defend a food boundary.

4. Forced conversations around diet and health, even if it is not directed at you.

What can you control?

You can control:

- Your choices and actions.

- How to react or respond to others.

- How you see yourself, and how you treat yourself.

- Who you spend time with.
- What social media groups and people you see.

You can't control:

- How other people react or behave.
- Other people's thoughts and perceptions of you (you don't even know what these truly are most of the time).
- What other people post on social media.

You are worthy of setting and having your own boundaries. You decide how your life is going to go, and you deserve to feel respected by those close to you. You can walk away from situations and conversations that make you feel bad and undermine the healing work you are doing.

Commitment

Making no exceptions means making a commitment to your mental and physical health on a deep and abiding level. And yet, so many of us struggle to keep our word to both ourselves and others.

Does any of this sound familiar? You make New Year's resolutions that are broken by February 1st. You start a new diet, hobby, or activity only to give up a few days or weeks into the proceedings. You say you will be there at 7 p.m., but at 6:50 p.m., you are still at home and wondering if you even want to go. Or you always run late for anything you commit to.

There are a number of possibilities behind why this is. Perhaps you are secretly (or not so secretly) avoiding the issue, or you are absentminded, overly optimistic about your abilities, or just not that interested in the first place.

For any commitment to any pursuit to work, you need to really want to be doing the thing (values, personal importance, and priorities). You need to understand how to set habits, and you need to put support systems in place to help you, at least in the beginning. These are all skills we have already discussed.

Another element is training your brain, so its default setting becomes automatically keeping your word. Like a muscle, this ability can be built and strengthened over time. To do this, you need to start small, choose goals that are at least 50-percent motivational for you (or more), and be SMART with your words. SMART means that when you describe what it is you are going to do, you make it Specific, Measurable, Achievable, Realistic, and Time-framed.

An example would be choosing to take a 10-minute walk around the block at lunchtime every day. This goal is very specific. You know exactly what, when, and how you will achieve it. It is also so small an activity that it is hard to feel any inner resistance to it.

It does not matter what you pick to do at first, just so long as you choose something fairly easy for you to do, and then stick to it, no matter what. Over time, you can add complexity or increase the size of the task. The simple act of giving and then keeping your word starts to register in your subconscious. Your mind starts waking up and saying, "Hey, when they say they will do a thing, it gets done."

Over time, this creates a new program in your subconscious, and it starts building your inner belief that you do what you say. And then later, when you do want to achieve a bigger goal, this program automatically supports the new commitment.

Your brain is like, "You usually do what you say, so why should this time be any different?"

Develop Mental Strength

By working on self-awareness, watching your negative inner voice, and reframing it, watching for faulty thinking, and working on healing any pain you have, you are already becoming stronger and more resilient.

Add an understanding of how to process and manage moods, and how to stay mindful and focus on your goals, and you level up even faster.

We all know that when you focus your attention on a thing, your energy and efforts will also be directed there. So, if you habitually focus on unhappy memories or thoughts, you tend to think yourself into depression or anxiety. If you focus on what you can't have, and what is wrong with the present moment, you might find a lot of anger and frustration energy building up. Likewise, if you turn your focus onto constructive thought and actions, these tend to be reinforced and supported.

This does not mean avoiding dealing with stuff. Feelings need to be noticed, named, and processed. Thoughts need to be observed and questioned. Problems need action plans and solutions. However, once this has been done, to keep focusing on the original issue is a bit like poking at a wound, putting extra bacteria in there, and never letting it heal.

This all makes sense, but how do we control where we focus?

Again, learning to manage your focus and attention is a learned skill. We are all told to concentrate or focus as kids, but sadly nobody really teaches us how. We also live in a highly distracted society, on our social media, multi-tasking, and so on. We practice distraction, and so we become good at that.

Instead of practicing distraction, try practicing focus in one of the following ways:

1. Mindfulness, which is simply just paying as much attention as possible to what is happening right now, in front of you. You can build your mindfulness muscle by simply representing yourself to the moment as often as possible. Use screensavers or reminders to help you do so. Practice sensory focus by immersing yourself in the moment using all your senses. Mindful eating would be savoring each bite, chewing slowly, noticing the texture and taste, and taking your time to look at the food, smell it, before cutting each bite and putting it in your mouth. Mindful presence can be applied in a similar way to any activity. Slow down, notice what you can see, hear, taste, smell, and feel.

2. Meditation is not only good for lowering stress levels, but it also helps train our brains to become super focused while remaining ultra-calm. This does not need to be a complicated process, with uncomfortable poses, strange mantras, and men in loincloths. Simply sitting quietly for a few minutes, in a comfortable position, with your eyes open and fixed on one point in front of you and breathing and counting each breath will do the trick. If your mind wanders, which it will, simply bring it back gently to focusing on the breath and start counting again from one if you have lost your place. The

counting is reflexive (you don't need to think about it that much), and with time, you will find the process gets easier. It's best to meditate with your eyes open, as you are training your brain to be focused and relaxed in life.

Guided meditation, or using a picture, mandala, or candle as the focal point is also helpful. You can find many great guided meditations on YouTube for free. You can also use any repetitive activity as part of a meditation. Washing the dishes? Do it mindfully, and slowly, focusing your mind on the warm, soapy water and how each dish slowly emerges from the grime. Walking? Focus on each footstep and notice how the ground feels beneath your feet.

In a fairly short time, you will not only feel calmer and generally more focused in life, but you will also find it easier to commit to and complete tasks and goals, too.

Building mental strength in all these ways will help you with your weight management and self-healing journey. You don't just commit, apply self-discipline, and remain super self-controlled magically and overnight. This is all a process, and only by understanding how your mind and body work together and using as many of the tools and tricks in this book as you can, will you make the consistent and permanent progress you desire.

Chapter 7: Step 6—Eat Healthily

Having a good grasp on your mental state, and building mental strength and self-discipline are all the building blocks of overcoming food addictions and emotional eating. What you also need is a practical and simple approach to what food you choose to eat, and what you do not.

Understanding some simple science behind what foods you align with, and also how to best eat them to maximize the weight management benefits will go a long way to supporting you on your journey. Not only will your weight and health steadily improve, but your overall mood, too. As you go, the need for junk food, sugars, salt, and fats will also gradually decrease until it becomes a lot easier to resist these urges.

Ready for it? Let's go.

What Is a Healthy Diet?

There are many great diet plan options out there that ascribe to the basics of healthy eating. I won't say any are better than the other, wrong, or right. It's more about what works for you and fits into your lifestyle.

Whatever eating plan you choose, make sure that it adheres to these basic nutritional guidelines, and you can't go too far wrong.

Go for More Low-Calorie Density

Low-calorie density means that pound for pound the food has a lower calorie count than other foods. These foods still have the same bulk, or amount, though. They are mostly made up of water and fiber, as well as other healthy nutrients, and all of this together means you are satisfied and feel full, while keeping your calorie count lower.

For example, a pound of fresh tomatoes has a calorie count of 90, compared to a pound of bagels that sit at 1,200 calories.

Do you see the difference?

Low-calorie-density foods include most vegetables and salad greens, fruits, cooked whole grains, oatmeal, and cooked beans and legumes. You can also put non-fat dairy here. Broth-based soups and non-fat fruit or vegetable smoothies are great choices. They fill you up and keep those hefty calories down.

High-calorie-density foods tend to be drier (i.e., contain less water content) and fattier. These include animal fats and proteins, dairy, nuts, seeds, bread, cereals, eggs, dried fruit, and oils. This does not make these foods bad, but what it does mean is that you need to limit your portions. Around 90-percent of your daily diet should be chosen for low-calorie foods. This will help bring down cholesterol, stabilize blood sugar, and lose excess weight, too. Pick only a few foods from the high calorie list and keep the total of these less than 4 ounces, if you can (Killoran, n.d.).

Go for Variety

Choose from red, yellow, green, and even blue foods, and mix it up as much as possible. Go for a rainbow on your plate. And yes, you do get blue food. Think about blueberries or blue corn.

Then, make sure you are also going for a healthy mix of the various food types and groups. Your body and brain even need some sugar and fats, but it is the type and amount that you need to be aware of.

If you think about the low versus high-calorie-density we just spoke about, you will know exactly what is meant by limiting certain food types.

Choose from whole grains like brown bread, pasta, and brown rice. I never could get my head around this, but once I tried it out, I found I loved the taste. Polenta and quinoa are also great choices.

Also add in legumes, nuts, seeds, leafy greens, and vegetables including potatoes, carrots, zucchini, sweet potatoes, broccoli, Brussels sprouts, corn, cucumbers, green beans, onions, peas, spinach, tomatoes, and so on. There is so much variety to delight your taste buds here. Just remember, nuts and seeds need to be limited if you are trying to lose weight, even if they are really healthy foods.

You can include low-sugar fruits like bananas, lemons, limes, kiwis, avocados, and berries, but consider limiting the fruits high in fructose like watermelons, dried fruits, pineapples, fruit juices, mangoes, cherries, apples, oranges, or very ripe bananas if you are watching weight and sugar levels. The sugars in fruit are not free sugars like in many processed foods, and don't have that much of an impact on blood sugar levels.

Low or nonfat dairy, eggs, and cheese such as cottage cheese are all fine. As are any nut milk products. Other cheeses, butter, and so on, are not bad foods, but do need to be limited from a calorie perspective if you are trying to manage your weight.

Animal proteins should be lean cuts, with a preference for chicken, turkey, and fish, which are all leaner, less fatty, and contain more healthy fats. Sadly, this does mean you need to ditch the strip of fat on your beef steak, let someone else eat your chicken skin, and avoid lard. Fat is one of the things that makes food tasty, so if you are avoiding or limiting it, you may need to jazz up your food with herbs and spices instead.

Cut Out Processed, Salty, Fatty, and Sugary Foods

There are many strange-sounding chemical names on the side of a food packet that are mostly harmless to humans, so don't get scared off by scientific lists of ingredients. Some food needs to be processed to make it safe for our consumption, like dairy, which is pasteurized to remove bacteria. Other foods, like seed oils, or olives, need to be processed so we can actually use them for purposes like cooking and eating. We couldn't generally do that in their raw state.

Minimally processed stuff, like chopped vegetables, roasted nuts, or bagged spinach are not a train smash. Although, for the highest nutritional value, it is best to do your chopping and peeling right before cooking. However, not all of us have the time for that.

Some processing, like frozen or canned goods with no chemical additives, actually locks in nutritional goodness.

I am talking more about foods processed with added ingredients. These are often ready-to-eat foods, and if you flip them over and check the labels, there will be a long list of ingredients that all sound a bit strange.

In general, as we don't all know what each thing is, and there are a lot of chemicals added to preserve shelf life, flavor, and the look and structure of the product, we can end up with a chemical storm in our bodies.

Remember that our bodies didn't have these additives a few hundred years ago, and they are not really set up to process them well. They can cause allergic reactions, digestive upsets, and even nervous disorders, because our bodies aren't set up to digest this stuff, so it often just gets stored in our fat deposits.

Moreover, most processed foods have extra salt, sugar, and fats added for flavor, and this is a no-go if you are trying to be healthy and manage weight. Also, some additives have been found to be downright bad for us. Countries can ban a certain additive, only to find it appears under a different name later. Those food manufacturers are so clever.

Processed foods include many breakfast cereals, health and energy bars, and drinks, tinned goods, chips, pies, processed meats like sausages, burgers, salami and pate, cakes, biscuits, and ready-made meals. Just because a product says 'healthy,' 'diet,' or something similar, does not mean it is.

Read the labels. The ingredients are usually listed in order of amount, so the first few will be the highest amounts. Look out for added sugar and salt (sodium).

Added sugar can hide behind words like glucose, cane sugar, corn syrup, maltose, dextrose, maltodextrin, lactose, fruit juice concentrate, molasses, honey, fructose, raw sugar, barley malt, treacle, and caramel.

When you read a label, you need to look at the serving size (and the number of servings in the pack), total calories per serving, and ingredients list. Avoid anything with added MSG (monosodium glutamate), trans fats, food dyes, sodium nitrate/nitrite, butylated hydroxyanisole (BHA), and butylated hydroxytoluene (BHT), sulfur dioxide, and potassium bromate (Mercola, 2010).

Don't forget to check your herb and spice labels, too. Go for single-state herbs and spices or your straightforward herbs or curry powders mixed from pure base spices, rather than complex spice mixes that invariably have MSG or something similar added. You should recognize everything on the label, and it should be an herb or spice, rather than an additive.

Honestly, I just think it is easier to choose fresh, raw, or homemade foods over all the processed stuff, because your body is more able to process it.

Don't Forget to Hydrate

Our bodies are mostly made up of water and liquids, and we need to keep topping this up, or like a swimming pool or fish tank, we will eventually clog up, and run dry.

We need water for all our cells to function. It helps get rid of waste, flushing out toxins via perspiration, urination, and bowel movements. It regulates body temperature, lubricates your joints, and protects sensitive tissue like eyes, mouth, and so on.

Dehydration can cause headaches, aches and pains, constipation, fatigue, dizziness, and confusion, increase the risk of kidney stones and lethargy. The worse it gets, the worse you get, and consistent or severe dehydration can be fatal.

So, we need to make darn sure we are hydrating, and we need to choose the right kinds of liquids to hydrate with. For our body's purposes, the simpler the better.

Water, hopefully from a pure source and not full of processing and cleaning chemicals, is always the best. Consider getting a good water purifier for your kitchen. The guideline is around 125 fluid ounces for adult men, and 91 fluid ounces for adult women. It sounds like a lot, but you get about 20-percent of this from your food, and the rest from everything that you drink, not just those glasses of water (Mayo Clinic, 2020).

Your best bet to ensure good hydration is to drink when you feel thirsty. If you are active, pregnant, breastfeeding, or ill, you may need to drink more. Around eight glasses a day is the general guideline, but you also need to let your body guide you. I make a point of drinking a glass of water before every meal or snack; before, during, and after exercise; and I also carry bottled water with me on the go.

If you seldom feel thirsty, and your urine is light yellow or colorless, you are on the right track. There is an issue where you can drink too much water, called hyponatremia, but this is often found mostly with athletes who force water during intense or lengthy exercise (Mayo Clinic, 2020).

In any event, what you choose to hydrate with should be plain water, or with added fresh lemon juice or a dash of fresh fruit juice or crushed berries. Soda water is also a great choice, and you can add some pizazz with a slice of lemon or orange, or some crushed mint leaves. Herbal teas or plain coffee, no milk or sugar added, and broth-based soups are also great ways to quench your thirst.

Avoid sugary sodas, sports, and energy drinks. Even those flavored waters have added sugar and additives. Sodas are high in calories and may quench your thirst but do nothing for your waistline. The high-sugar content packs in the calories, but you remain hungrier than before. And we all know the story about additives already, right?

Aim to Stay Fuller Longer

This is mainly for weight-management purposes. You have two main hormones in your body regulating your hunger.

Leptin, made by your fat cells, tells you to stop eating. Ghrelin is released as your belly empties, signaling your body that more food is needed. It makes you hungry, basically.

Unfortunately, when you are overweight, you may find you have built up a resistance to leptin, as well as eating for emotional or pleasurable and sensory reasons that have nothing to do with actual hunger.

Ghrelin peaks and creates the feeling of hunger, and then subsides about 20 minutes after that first mouthful, as that is roughly how long it takes for the food to start filling your stomach and the body to realize it and stop releasing ghrelin. You then have around three hours or so before the cycle begins again.

The more fat you have stored, the more leptin you have available, which may have something to do with overweight people getting used to it and building resistance over time. Sleep also affects leptin levels, interestingly.

There are some cunning tricks you can use to fool your body into thinking it is not that hungry.

First, go for loads of liquid-based stuff. Drinking a glass of water about half an hour before a meal can help reduce your appetite significantly.

Broth-based soups, whether chunky or smooth, with loads of vegetables in them, will quickly travel to your stomach and fill up that space, as will low-fat dairy or vegetable-based smoothies. Juicing is definitely a master plan for weight control. You can still add to that with salads, whole grain bread or crackers, low or nonfat cottage cheese or spreads, or other healthy side snacks.

Proteins also help keep you fuller for longer, but the portion sizes need to be controlled.

Lastly, sleep is a big thing. if you are not sleeping well, you tend to be hungrier as a rule. Get your sleep routine right and get enough of it.

Food Preparation

It's all very well to choose all the right, healthy ingredients, but if we choose the wrong preparation methods, we are in effect wasting our time.

Lean meat fried in butter. Potatoes roasted in lard. Salads drizzled with creamy, processed salad dressing. Veggies stir-fried with oil or butter. Yes, these all sound delicious, but if this is what you're doing, you are missing the point.

We need to be lowering fat content, not adding to it. So that means grilling, baking, or steaming your food, rather than frying, deep-frying, or sautéing it. If you wish to allow yourself a teensy pad of butter on your baked potato, you do that as part of your high-calorie and fat portion control. It's better to start using flavorings like hummus, lemon juice, herbs, and spices, or even low-fat cottage cheese on that yummy potato.

Cook from Scratch

Cooking from fresh foods—slicing, peeling, and dicing—and still choosing the right cooking method and knowing which herbs and spices to use may sound like a real headache.

This is especially true if you have not cooked much before or have come to rely on ready-made meals.

There are a few things you can do to make it all easier.

First, buying frozen, pre-sliced, and peeled veggies is quite fine. I will even buy packs of freshly prepped vegetables and toss them in the freezer to preserve their nutritional content.

Choose one or two healthy meals and just focus on learning how to cook those. A baked potato, with some steamed veggies and a skinless chicken breast, takes a maximum of 30 minutes to make and very little effort. You can slowly build up your culinary skills.

You can even make a large portion of a meal and freeze what is left for another day. I don't like to eat the same meal twice in a row, but freezing a healthy brown pasta and vegetable, or a great curry and brown rice is not that difficult. Just make sure to label stuff, or you end up with a lot of surprise meals.

Alternatively, there are meal delivery and preparation services that have caught on to the fact that people want to eat more healthily. So, if you really have no time for meal prep, find a local food service that truly does make healthy food, and make sure you have enough freezer space. There are loads of home-based small businesses doing this kind of thing now.

Meal Planning

Some of us love to plan and others, not so much. However, in the early days of trying to get a handle on healthy eating, this is really your best friend.

It takes a few minutes to go online and check out the calories in a serving of some of your favorite healthy foods. If you have a calorie goal per day to maintain or lose weight, you then can create a basic meal plan for breakfast, lunch, dinner, and snacks, based on the list of foods you have researched.

What helped me was to list three or four options per mealtime. I could then also shop with that in mind, so I had all my ingredients to hand for the week.

These days, there are also a vast array of online sites and apps that will do all of this for you. They will even work out your recommended calorie intake, and supply meal plans, recipes, and ideas. Some even allow you to add things to a shopping list and then order online. So really, if you aren't a planner, there is no excuse now for not finding the right plan and using it.

Search for meal planning and ordering websites to see what is available, especially those that can order and deliver in your area if you are a busy bee and don't have time to shop, let alone cook. There are so many of these, and so many of them are really good, that I cannot list them all. Eatingwell.com was one I have used and enjoyed, but there are many others you can try out.

Some useful apps to try out are Noom, Mealtime, Make my Plate, Yummly, and more. Try them out until you find one that suits you. Many of them also let you share recipes with family and friends, which is helpful when these people are open to supporting your diet and cooking in line with what you need at social events.

Don't forget that meal planning also means making sure that you have healthy snacks on hand whenever you need them, and that you make sure you eat before your hunger levels go past the danger zone, where you just binge on anything you can find. That defeats the purpose of mindful, healthy eating. So being prepared is key.

Healthy and quick snack ideas include pre-packed bags or lunch boxes of popcorn; vegetable sticks and hummus, or cottage cheese as a dip; kale chips; dark chocolate; nuts and trail mix; low-fat yogurt with mixed berries; apple and peanut butter, cucumber or tomato slices with hummus or cottage cheese, hard-boiled eggs, olives, whole grain crackers or sandwiches, or even just a piece of fruit.

My favorite trick is packing last night's leftovers in a lunch box to go.

Portion Control

We've mentioned that you should go for 90-percent of your intake based on low-calorie-density foods. However, there are other considerations, too.

Your meal plans and calorie goals may have already given you some idea, but to keep things really simple, consider the following guide per day.

Aim for two to three cups of vegetables, one to two cups of fruit, around five to eight ounces of whole grains, a maximum of three cups of nonfat or low-fat dairy, a maximum of five ounces of protein (for example, nuts, seeds, and some legumes), and around five teaspoons worth of healthy oils like pure olive oil, flaxseed, avocado, walnut, sesame, or grapeseed oils.

Bear in mind that an ounce is roughly the same size as your outstretched thumb, or a handful if you can't be bothered to measure stuff. A cup can be equated to your fist in size. The size of your palm is around three ounces of protein. The tip of your thumb equates to about a teaspoon. This is a very rough guideline as obviously our hand sizes vary quite a bit. So, you may need to take the time to measure out your favorite foods in ounces or cups at least once, to get a visual idea of portion sizes.

You may need to adjust these amounts based on your calorie goals and weight loss targets.

You can use the plate-by-plate method as well, where each plate is half veggies or fruit; a quarter of complex carbs like whole grains, brown rice, pasta, or potato; and whatever protein amount you have left in your daily allowance.

Avoid added sugars. Rather, use one of the healthy sweetener alternatives we mentioned earlier, or cut sugar out altogether. Choose spices and herbs, rather than adding extra salt to your food, although, this is more for general health than weight loss. Sodium does affect how much water your body retains but does not really influence fat content. Only a healthy eating approach does that.

Eating Out

As consciousness grows around healthier eating, we find lots of options more readily available for us.

Take a look at health-focused restaurants in your area. Some will openly advertise as being green, vegan, healthy, gluten-free, and so on. Choose these as eating-out options when possible.

If you don't get that choice and know ahead of time where you will be eating, you can check out their menu to see what fits in with your diet plan, and even contact the restaurant in advance with any special requests.

You know what healthy eating is now, so quickly scanning a menu to find meals that exclude unhealthy chemical additives (ask about MSG specifically), are freshly prepared, and also exclude white, processed flours, cheeses, and creamy sauces are not that difficult.

Go for broth-based soups, salads, grilled and baked foods, and leave off any batters or cream-based sauces.

You can ask for your burger without the bun or ask if they have any whole wheat bread options, request that they leave off any creamy sauces, and even ask for extra vegetables. Most places are quite used to this by now. Even at pizza places, many offer a gluten-free base (which means it won't have processed flours), cauliflower or quinoa crusts, and you can order veggies on top and leave off the cheese or add on low-fat cheese options.

As a last resort, if you know you are going somewhere that has nothing that fits in with your new eating plan, simply pack and take a small lunch box. Explain to the restaurant and the social group that you have a sensitive stomach or can't eat the kinds of foods on the menu. Most people won't question you past that. If you get a particularly pushy or nosey person, you can just say you prefer not to go on about it, or that it is a really boring topic, and change topics. And you can still order drinks and ask for a plate for your pre-packed items.

Eating out at people's homes is a little trickier. If it is possible, have a quiet word with the host a few days before, so that they can provide for you. Make sure you serve for yourself and simply don't eat or don't serve anything that is not part of your plan. I know it is good manners to eat what is provided, but if you don't make a huge fuss about it, neither will your host. In fact, at many social gatherings, people don't even notice what you are doing, so skipping the cheese platter, and cutting off the fatty portions of your steak will mostly go unnoticed.

Good Mood Foods and Supplements

As we now understand, behind food addiction, there often sit emotional challenges. It does not hurt to adapt our diet a little to help and support us in dealing with these bad feelings.

Some foods are known to boost and help stabilize a better mood, and that can only help you in your fight to conquer your addiction. When you are feeling a bit down, instead of turning to the usual comfort foods like pizzas, burgers, chips, cakes, and biscuits, consider trying out one of these mood boosters. And if you are feeling constantly anxious, low, or out of sorts, make sure they are a regular part of your diet.

- Omega-3 fatty acids include DHA (docosahexaenoic acid) and EPA (eicosapentaenoic acid). Both substances are strongly linked to reducing inflammation in the brain and promoting neurogenesis (new brain cells), and more neural connections. All of this helps with mood, as well as memory and focus, too. Eating walnuts, chia seeds, flaxseed, and plant oils like soybean and canola all help with Omega 3 levels. Supplementing with Omega 3s in capsule form is also a great idea. Just make sure that the EPA level sits at a minimum of 1,000 mg, and don't go above 5 g of Omega 3 per day. If you are on any anticoagulant medications, chat with your doctor before supplementing with extra Omega 3s as well (NIH, 2021). In general, Omega 3s are also helpful for reducing dry eye and mouth disorders, arthritis, ADHD, heart health, and for promoting great-looking skin, hair, and nails. What's not to like?

- Fermented foods that promote gut health are top of the pops. Gut health is super important for mood management. An inflamed gut directly influences levels of tolerance, irritability, focus, and general resilience. It is also directly linked with increased allergies and poor immune response. We often refer to our gut as a second brain, and researchers have even found neurons present in the gut. Things like sugars and chemical additives inflame our guts, so if we can cut those out, and feed our digestive system with gut-healthy foods to support it, we can make a big difference to our quality of life. Foods like kimchi, live yogurt, kefir, sauerkraut, and kombucha all provide good bacteria that we need present in our guts for gut health and digestion. Supplementing with pre- and probiotics is also a good idea. Not only does it ensure a happier gut, but it also helps strengthen your immune system, too.

- Dark chocolate, in moderation, is a pleasurable and healthy treat. It's high in flavonoids that reduce brain inflammation, increase blood flow to the brain and generally help with good brain function, which in turn helps stabilize mood. Limit it to one or two squares a day, or as a special treat every now and then.

- Bananas and berries are great mood boosters. Vitamin B6 in bananas helps synthesize feel-good chemicals in the body, and the fiber and natural sugars also provide a lovely slow release of energy. Bananas, especially slightly greener ones, are also full of prebiotics to support a strong gut microbiome. Berries, rich in antioxidants, anthocyanins, and phenols, are also helpful for brain health. Go for the dark reds, blues, and purple berries, and if you can't find them fresh, keep a pack of frozen berries, and add a handful to your smoothies. If you mix frozen berries, banana, and low-fat yogurt you get a delightful ice-cream alternative, too. Even frozen bananas on their own, blended and refrozen for a bit, make a healthy sweet treat.

- Oats, especially steel-cut, which are higher in fiber, are whole grains rich in iron. The fiber helps slow digestion, giving you a healthy, slow release of energy, as well as helping you feel fuller for longer.

- Nuts and seeds are also good for your mood. They are a high-calorie density food, so you do need to limit the portions, but including them with your salads, oats porridge, or smoothies is a great way to provide your body with tryptophan, and thus help produce more feel-good hormones. Go for almonds, cashews, peanuts, walnuts, pumpkin seeds, sesame, and sunflower seeds. Nuts and seeds also contain other trace vitamins and minerals which help peak brain function, like zinc and selenium.

- Lentils and legumes like chickpeas, peas, kidney beans, black beans, soybeans, pinto beans, edamame, and navy beans are all good choices. They are high in vitamin B, which increases levels of helpful neurotransmitters and feel-good hormones. Trace elements of zinc, selenium, magnesium, and iron also boost your mood.

- Finally, caffeine helps with mood management, within reason, because too many cups of java will give you the jitters, too. Everything in balance, but the adenosine (which helps cell energy transfer) in caffeine helps increase alertness and focus. It also increases mood-boosting brain transmitters like dopamine. Coffee, green tea, or cocoa, without added milk and sugar, is your best source of natural caffeine. The FDA (US Food and Drug Administration) cites 400 mg per day as the maximum amount recommended. That's about four or five cups.

(Davidson, 2020)

Benefits of Veganism for Weight Loss

Going meatless is not everyone's idea of a fun time, but it definitely is a fast way to lower cholesterol, lose weight, and generally boost mood and general health.

Going vegan does not just mean cutting out meat. It also means no eggs, dairy, fish, gelatin, or any food or food product that comes from animals. Vegans make this choice for a variety of reasons, from health, through to helping reduce the impact on climate change, lowering food bills, weight loss, and also out of an affinity for animals. Mass production of animal food products is known for its less than ideal treatment of the animals. There are certainly groups that attempt to farm more ethically and slaughter more humanely, but in the end, being killed for your meat, bred endlessly for your milk, and being kept often caged for your entire life is not a nice way to go. And as we mentioned, there's the effect of increased methane produced by the thousands of herds of cows, sheep, goats, and so on, which increases global warming. So, there's a lot of reasons to consider a vegan diet.

This is probably not something you could do overnight, but you could slowly move toward it over time to make the choice stick.

I drink only oat milk for added calcium and water, and while this may sound like I am depriving myself, once I made the choice, I never looked back. Not only does it mean my weight stays under control, but my general health, mood, and energy levels are better than they have ever been before.

A vegan diet, if approached properly, is known to be richer in essential nutrients like fiber, plant compounds, antioxidants, and vitamins and minerals such as potassium, folate, magnesium, and vitamins C, A, and E. They are ironically actually higher iron than meat-based diets, although plant irons aren't as absorbable for humans.

It is advisable to consider supplementing with iron, B vitamins, zinc, and calcium if you are unsure that you are getting enough from your diet.

Because the foundation of a vegan diet contains mainly low-calorie-density foods, you do lose weight faster. It also cuts out all animal fats, which means your cholesterol regulates more easily. Blood sugar levels also appear to regulate, and your kidney function improves, too. Heart disease risks are reduced, because not only is your cholesterol lower, but all those fresh fruits and vegetables and extra fiber, support healthy heart function.

Whole food, plant-based diets also reduce general inflammation, which assists brain function, as well as reduces pain for arthritis-sufferers, and helps us with aches and pains in general (Petre, 2021).

If you are considering moving across to a vegan approach, you would want to ensure you are getting enough, as well as a variety, of the foods you need to support good health. People are omnivores, which means that our bodies can process animal as well as plant-based food. However, even with this in mind, the amount of protein humans ate in the wild was far less than what we deluge our bodies with these days. Back then, a few eggs, grubs, small birds, and insects would have made up the usual protein source, and occasionally meat from a larger hunt, but that was not a daily occurrence. We ate way more seeds, nuts, fruits, whole grains, and vegetables, as these were easier to find or grow.

Eating healthily as a vegan means that you:

- Base your meals on whole grains like potatoes, brown and seed bread, pasta, rice, or other starchy carbohydrates.

- Choose dairy alternatives like soy, or nut milk, and yogurts. Almond, oat, coconut, and hemp seed milk are readily available in most supermarket chains and health shops these days. Tofu-based foods can be very tasty.

- Go for at least five portions of fruit and vegetables daily and mix it up as much as possible by choosing from a wider variety of these foods. Good sources of plant-based iron are green, leafy vegetables like broccoli, watercress, and spinach.

- Add legumes, nuts, seeds, pulses, and beans to your food for added plant-based protein. Lentils and rice provide a complete protein all by themselves.

- Add healthy, unsaturated oils to your meals. Sesame seeds and sesame seed oils are especially good for you, and delicious. A dash of truffle oil will make any dish spark with that umami yumminess.

- Yeast extract, like Marmite, is delicious on whole grain toast, and a good source of vitamin B12.

- Make sure you get enough sunshine or supplement with vitamin D if you feel that you don't.

(NHS, 2018)

Being vegan does not mean you can't eat sugary foods that have no animal-based ingredients in them, but as we know how bad sugar is for our guts, inflammation, our brains, and our calorie goals, it is best to stay mindful and not fall into that trap. Therefore, it is best to slowly replace foods over time, rather than cut out all sugars, processed food, and animal-based foods all at once.

If you rush any new eating plan, you might create a deprivation mindset, where all you can think about is what you can't eat. And as you know, where your attention goes, your focus grows, until eventually, that is all you can think about. Instead, take an "I choose" or "I can have" mindset, where you are clear on what you can have and that is where you keep your focus. Finding sweet treats like banana ice cream, dark chocolate, fruits, and so on, to replace the cakes, cookies, and sugary sweets is a good idea. And there are loads of sugar-free products in stores, as well as vegan and sugar-free treats to be found in recipe ideas online. Build up a few of these and make sure you delight your taste buds often enough with them that you don't start longing for all the wrong stuff again.

All these healthy eating suggestions can sound like a lot to do all at once. And it is better to not try to change too much overnight. Go back to our section on creating and maintaining good habits. Use those methods to slowly cut out the unhealthy stuff and introduce healthy options that you can like.

It is better to make slower progress, that you can stick to, than try to change the world all at once and relapse a few days later, because it is too hard.

The thing about self-discipline is that it, like a muscle, strengthens slowly and with lots of help. For example, when I first stopped sugar in my coffee, I started slowly. For a week or two, I dropped from three teaspoons to two, and then to one. After a month of that, I dropped to none and then started drinking my coffee black with no sugar at all. My taste buds slowly acclimatized, and now, as I mentioned earlier, I drink water or dairy-free milk only. However, my process was slow, but consistent progress, with no going back. That helped my weight and my self-discipline, too.

Healthy Eating Tricks

Over and above, it's important to know what to eat and why there are some ingenious weight-management tips and tricks you can try to help you along.

Eat Slower and Stop Sooner

As we know, it takes some time for your brain to register that you are full. By eating more slowly, you give that whole process a chance to catch up.

This also feeds into mindful eating, such as cutting your food, chewing more slowly, and savoring each bite; and pausing in between each mouthful to perhaps take a swig of water or tea as well. Although our lives can be very busy, taking extra few minutes to mindfully eat your meal is just so much better for you on a mental, emotional, and physical level.

The other thing to try is to stop eating before you feel fully sated. You can leave those last few bites and donate them to the family pet instead, or the compost heap. Or simply stop eating a few minutes before you normally would. You know that in a short while, you will feel fully sated as your mind catches up with your body.

Eat When Hungry, Stop When You Aren't

It sounds so simple, but if you are sensitive enough to your body's hunger cues, simply let it tell you when to eat. I find that sticking to set mealtimes can sometimes make you eat more than you need. You think, "Oh well, it is lunchtime, so I might as well eat something." However, in fact, at that time, you don't really need to, you just do it, because someone said regular meals are important. They are, but it is better to let your body tell when exactly 'regular' is. Your body knows when it is time to top up.

Just make sure to keep a healthy meal or snack at the ready so when you start to feel a bit hungry, you don't turn to junk food.

Plate it Up, on Smaller Plates

Rather than grabbing handfuls of food on the fly, try always putting your meal on a plate. Yes, this does create extra dishes to wash, but it also serves to help you stay mindful of the amounts you are eating, and how you are balancing the various food groups as well.

Moreover, as we get older, or our activity levels change, we may need to adjust our portion sizes. I don’t need to eat as much as I did when I was 15, 25, or even 30. Realizing that it was a simple matter to reduce my portion sizes, I found I was just as full and energized as ever. Before, I had just been eating the same amount as what Mom dished up for me when I was a kid. I hadn't stopped to question it.

Also, if you get clever and use smaller bowls and plates, you tend to serve less for yourself anyway. The eye and brain are partially fooled into thinking you are still eating more than you actually are.

Out of Sight, Out of Mind

Don't stock up on junk foods. Or, if you are sharing a home with those who eat unhealthy stuff, create a space or cupboard that is just yours, and never go into the other food storage. That way, if you aren't seeing unhealthy choices, you are way less likely to make them.

Reduce your Alcohol Intake

An average glass of dry wine can cost you a quarter of your calorie allowance. And how often do we stick to just one?

This can seriously affect your waistline, not to mention your mood. While at first, alcohol relaxes you, and removes inhibitions, too much makes you reckless, uncoordinated, and can result in memory loss and all kinds of other health and safety issues. Alcohol continues to affect you into the next day, and the raised sugar levels, raised heart rate, dehydration, and depressant function of alcohol can mimic symptoms of anxiety and depression.

Stay Hydrated

The more broth-based soups, smoothies, and other healthy liquids you pump into your system the better. Not only do you hydrate better this way, but you feel fuller for longer, and less inclined to snack or binge on junk foods.

Drinking before a meal also signals your body that you are fuller sooner, so it helps you eat less.

So now you know what a healthy diet is, you are free to experiment with a version that suits you. There are many diet plans and options that work well, and you may find one of them appeals to you or fits in with your lifestyle better than the others. I will take you through a few of the more popular ones a bit later.

Take some time to surf the internet and find easy-to-cook, and simple, fast recipes that fit into your eating plan. Find some recipes for tasty snacks and treats, too. Keep them readily accessible for when you plan your shopping and cook your meals. I find it helps to always keep a premade tasty snack in the fridge. This stops me from impulse buying and eating.

Use Aromatherapy

Burning a vanilla-scented candle during dinner has been known to help reduce hunger. Perhaps the sweet scent is enough that you can more easily skip dessert. Most essential oils can't directly reduce your weight, but they can improve mood, and, as we know, that does affect weight management. Any oils that reduce anxiety and assist with inflammation are useful.

Lavender is a mood booster and calmative. It also helps with digestion and sleep.

Lemon oil is detoxifying and regenerative, as well as energizing.

Grapefruit oil helps detox and regulate blood sugar.

Peppermint oil is energizing and anti-inflammatory.

Bergamot, clary sage, and ylang-ylang are also very calming and restorative.

(West Rosenthal, 2016)

Essential oils are not generally to be taken internally. They are used in an oil burner or rubbed into your belly button or the base of your feet, or simply used as a massage oil. A few drops of the oil in about 20 ml of a base or carrier oil are sufficient for these purposes, but if in any doubt, consult an aromatherapist. Also, some oils are dangerous to use around animals, or if you are pregnant or breastfeeding.

Morning Coffee

Starting your day with a cup of java taken either black or with a dash of non-fat milk suppresses appetite. You tend to eat less and need to eat later, than if you don't have that cup.

Color Up

Serve your food on plates in a contrasting color. It creates a mental, conscious, and visible reminder of the amount you are serving. So, eating your pasta on a red or blue plate, or your meat on a green plate might help reduce portion sizes. Eat your salads in a green bowl or on a green plate to eat more of those.

Chew, Chew, Chew

If your hunger levels aren't that great, or you are just feeling bored, chew some sugar-free gum. It gives you something to do, has a flavor, and distracts you from the eating urge.

Ultimately, you need to add as many tricks to your repertoire as you can, because you will find a few that really stick, and make enough of a difference. All you need is just enough to stop you from reaching out for that unhealthy food option.

Chapter 8: Holistic Weight Loss

There's a lot more to weight control than just diet and exercise. As we have already seen, especially with food addiction, it has a lot to do with self-awareness, healing, and mood management, too.

Not only that, but there are even further things you can put in place that will support you during your weight loss journey. Beating food addiction is no small accomplishment, and you really need all the help you can get, especially in the early days.

Approaching the issue from every angle is your best bet.

These are tried-and-tested ways to build your resilience and support consistent weight management.

Sleep

Getting a decent night's sleep is more important to weight loss than many people realize. When you are tired, you have a reduced capacity to make good eating choices. It's easier to grab that burger or have that extra latte, because you can justify it by saying you are too tired to do more.

It's also easier to skip your exercise routine and be a lazy person.

Your tolerance for stress and problems is way less, your moods swing about all over the place, and that is a perfect environment for food addiction to flourish in. A dull frontal lobe means you simply can't make decisions or practice self-control the same way when you are fatigued.

Your brain's reward centers also seem to light up when you are overtired, and that means you are even more likely to binge eat, overeat, or eat the wrong things. Tired people snack more, late at night, and tend to crave high-carb snacks. The University of Chicago ran a study that showed sleep-deprived people ate snacks with double the fat content, compared to the well-rested group (WebMD, n.d.).

Not enough sleep also increases cortisol, the stress hormone, and that makes your body conserve energy and burn fat more slowly, too. Your ability to regulate insulin decreases as well, which means your blood sugar levels become more unstable, affecting mood and food cravings.

When you sleep more, you make less ghrelin, which is the hunger chemical. Your brain and body use this time to detox and get rid of any buildup of waste. You also use the REM (rapid eye movement) dream state to sort through the day's events, and in a way, this is a kind of defragmentation and hard-drive cleanup for the brain, too.

Your body and muscles rest and your energy replenishes. And your RMR (resting metabolic rate) goes up, too, the more you sleep. This means that you burn more calories even when lying down or sitting still.

In short, sleep is pretty important for weight management.

Sadly, so many people battle with getting a good night's sleep. Some of what I am about to suggest will be a no-brainer for you, but make sure you are addressing all the good sleep criteria before complaining that nothing works. Like puzzle pieces, all these factors add up to good sleep, and one missing piece means the picture is incomplete.

1. Level up your sleep environment. Make sure your pillows and mattress are breathable and comfortable. Invest in soft sheets and cozy blankets. Is your sleepwear loose-fitting and comfortable? Block out light and noise with blackout curtains, white noise, soundproofing, or even comfy earplugs. Curtains, carpets, and wall-hangings all help reduce noise, too. What about the room temperature? If it is hot, get a fan and use a bug screen or herbal spray to keep mosquitoes away. If it is chilly, all you really need are warm blankets.

2. Make sure you are moving around enough during the day, so your body feels at least a little physically tired by sleep time.

3. Are you getting enough sunshine? Your body needs this to regulate and produce the hormones which both wake you up and help you sleep. If you don't have much access to natural light, consider buying a UVA/UVB bulb for your office or regular living space.

4. Keep away from late-night snacks. If you'd like to eat within two hours of bedtime, keep meals light, like a fruit salad, or some whole grain toast and soup. Alcohol and caffeine should be on your no-go list a good few hours before you plan to sleep. Also, too much sugar and junk food during the day will also interfere with a good rest.

5. Get your sleep routine right. You decide the best combination of things to do that works for you. Definitely stop screen time and any hectic mental

activity at least 30 minutes before bedtime and consider getting a blue-light filter for your screens to stop them from messing with your melatonin (a hormone which has long been associated with control of the sleep–wake cycle) production. A warm bath or shower helps you feel comfortable and clean and provides a relaxing cool-down period right before bed. Some light yoga or stretching, especially lying with your feet up against a wall for a bit, is also very relaxing. And lastly, get your stresses and worries out by doing some journaling, and reflecting on the day. Planning for tomorrow's events may also help some people relax and let go of some anxiety.

6. Natural sleep supplements might be handy, especially if you need to reprogram a good sleep habit. Believe me, sleep or the lack of sleep can be habituated. Supplements like valerian, melatonin, chamomile, l-theanine, and magnesium can all help with better sleep. Remember to consult a professional before taking any medication.

7. Some meditation, belly breathing, or sound therapy using MHz on a timer that stops playing after an hour or so is all useful. YouTube has plenty of MHz for relaxation and sleep.

8. If you find yourself waking up often, use a sleep reset. These are really simple to do. You must not under any circumstances touch your phone, play a game, use your computer, or watch TV. Get out of bed, sit somewhere dimly lit, and quiet, and maybe read, journal, meditate or just sip a warm beverage. Once you start feeling sleepy again, go back to bed.

If you have tried all the above, and applied your knowledge of habit setting, and you still aren't sleeping, get yourself checked out for sleep apnoea or some other possible physical cause for the problem. Be careful what medication you take, as some sleeping tablets paralyze the muscles or delete your memory, but don't actually make you sleep as such. Others leave you groggy the next day, and neither of these are great results. Ask your physician about this, as well as how long it takes to work, how long it stays in your system, and how addictive the pill might be (Domingues, 2006). Sometimes, all you need is to use them for a short period to help you get back into a good sleep habit.

Get a Mentor

Much like any addict, having a special someone you can trust and respect to lean on occasionally helps a lot. The kind of person who makes a good mentor is someone with no personal agenda, and who has walked the food addiction path themselves so they can support you with empathy and kindness.

They need to be able to remind you that you are an addict, and how serious it will be if you lapse back into your addictive behavior.

The idea is that you both, by mutual agreement, commit to each other. This means that when you feel the urge to snack on junk food, have an extra glass of wine, or binge on anything at all, you can call them, and they will provide enough distraction and mentorship to help you avoid trouble and keep to your goals.

This can, and should, also include you being allowed and even encouraged to call when you are feeling anxious, depressed, or emotional, and you can't manage the feelings on your own. As we know, emotions underlie food addiction, so a mentor will understand that from time to time, you may just need someone neutral to talk to.

You may very well find such a person in a food addiction support group, or you may have a good friend who is willing to do this for you.

Access Your Subconscious Mind

Right, so you have a conscious mind. That is everything you are consciously aware of and deals with short-term memory. It is logical and analyzes whatever you experience. It is the decision-maker, and it is self-aware.

In many senses, it is the gatekeeper of your mind or the guard at the drawbridge. It is critical and analyzes everything before it is allowed entry into your subconscious.

Your subconscious mind is a huge recording device. It faithfully keeps track of whatever the conscious mind thinks and chooses to do. Long term memory sits in your subconscious. Once you access a specific memory, it comes back into your conscious mind for as long as you are focusing on it. The subconscious directly affects habitual behavior, your "inner voice", and is always paying attention and recording.

The subconscious works mainly with visuals and with emotions attached to whatever your recordings are. So, you can end up stuck with some pretty unhelpful habits, feelings, and behaviors based on whatever sits in your subconscious.

The good news is that you can overwrite unhelpful recordings, and bypass limiting beliefs and behaviors, by bypassing the conscious mind and going directly to the subconscious.

There are a few rules that apply to this whole system.

- Whatever you imagine is way more powerful than knowledge. For example, you might logically know that you are in no personal danger when watching a horror movie, but your imagination is sparked, and you still feel scared anyway. Reason always gives way to imagination.

- You can't internalize opposing beliefs or ideas. If your core belief is that honesty is important to you, if you tell a "white lie", you may find yourself experiencing a great deal of stress, no matter how you try to rationalize things to yourself. Once a concept has been accepted by your conscious mind as true, it will remain there until it can be replaced. Also, the longer an idea is held in the subconscious, the harder it is to replace.

- The more effort you put into consciously changing your subconscious mind, the smaller the result. For example, if you are battling to sleep based on subconscious worries or stress, no matter how much you try to force the issue, you can forget about a good night's sleep. The harder you try, the less effective your efforts.

- Every thought you have will cause a physical reaction in your body. We have seen this with our fears, and fight-freeze-flight responses. Too much anger stimulates your adrenal glands (these glands produce hormones that help regulate, among other things, response to stress) and leads to burnout. Too much worry appears to affect your gut and can lead to ulcers. Anxiety and fear put you on high alert, raising your blood pressure, sometimes dangerously or chronically.

Any thought that is highly emotional will record more strongly in your subconscious mind, as well.

So, what does all of this mean for you? Well, if you have a food addiction, it means that you will have a bunch of unhelpful recordings programmed into your subconscious that need replacing. It also means pure will-power or force will not do the trick.

We have already spoken about managing and processing thoughts and emotions, and dealing with that negative inner voice, but there are further tools you can add to your armory.

All of them bypass the conscious mind and sneak in past the guards into the castle of your subconscious so you can replace unhelpful ideas with ones that will be more supportive of your fight against food addiction.

Visualization

There are two ways to use visualization to access your subconscious. You can use both if you like. One is via a vision board, and the other is by using a recorded visualization script.

Practical Exercise: Create a Vision Board

Think about all your health and weight management goals and keep them in mind as you search the internet or flip through magazines. You are looking for visuals that show what it is you want.

Choose a few that really stand for what you want. Print them out in color and stick them all up in a collage on a big piece of A3 (or larger) cardstock paper.

Leave a little space in between images. In there, you will write words, such as short keywords that are also matched to your goals. However, make them specific. For example, "Fit to climb the stairs breathing easily", "At peace with myself", "Normal-range blood pressure", "Size [x]", or "Able to shop off the rack." Keep them in the present tense, as if you have already achieved them.

Take some time to really consider what these goals are. They will be linked to the reasons you want to beat the addiction.

Also, think about the emotions that will go with these things once you have achieved them. Things like, calm, happy, proud, disciplined, motivated, focused, peaceful, light, active, and excited. Pop these words in among the goal keywords and the images. Get as creative as you like, but it does not need to be a work of art, just meaningful to you and easy to read and see.

If you are good at this type of thing, you could even use the Canva app or create a digital board.

Stick the vision board somewhere you will see it as much as possible. I stuck mine up on the wall behind my laptop screen, so it had the chance to seep into my brain whenever I looked up from my work.

Scripted Visualizations

The same goals, keywords, and descriptions of feelings you came up with for your vision board can be used again for this. You can either keep it simple, and just lie quietly after meditation, after waking, or before bedtime. Close your eyes and visualize yourself at your ideal weight.

Make sure to be very clear in the vision. Describe as many senses and positive emotions as you can, too. What clothes are you wearing, where are you, what are you doing, and what do you look like all together. It helps to think about this as if it was a movie playing in your head, and then let the show unfold.

Alternatively, you can record your goals and happy feeling words on your phone, and again make it as sensory as possible. Write it out like a script for a movie and record it for playback before bed or after waking, or even both.

I found some great, pre-made scripts for healing, anxiety, sleep, and even body image, on a site called *Inner Health Studio*. There are similar sites out there that also have various options for visualization scripts if you don't want to make your own.

Mantras and Affirmations

Affirmation has been a buzzword for quite some time, but these often don't work, because we don't really understand fully how they work. It is not simply creating a list of things you would like. There is a very specific way to create affirmations that your subconscious can accept.

If you start out with wildly unbelievable statements, no part of your mind will fall for it, because at the root, you simply don't believe this thing is possible. Therefore, it does not really work.

You need to engage with your mind in ways that are both motivational and believable. For example, saying "I always get things right", could be replaced with, "Every day, I am getting better at [x]."

Affirmations need to be short, powerful, present tense, and attached to a positive emotion. That is the magic formula.

Practical Exercise: Create Your Affirmations

These will be short to medium-term desires that you have for your life. For the purposes of this book, we will keep them focused on mental and physical health and weight management. You can add others if you wish.

Write down your answers to the following:

1. What life area do you want to address now? Mental or physical?
2. What is your desired outcome, and how will you feel when you achieve this goal?
3. What has been stopping you from achieving this thing?

4. What will you do, think, be or feel that will help you get to your goal?
5. How can you stay motivated and connected to your goal?

Now, create around four or five short suggestions or statements that are positive, specific, simple, exciting, realistic, personal, and written in the present tense.

Avoid the words: try, no, not, don't, don't want, will, am going to, or anything similar. Any negative words like "I don't want" or "I won't" work exactly the opposite to your intention, as they simply focus your brain on the thing, and not the intention. Your brain filters out the "I don't" and all it sees is the thing you are trying to avoid and then records this. Then you get exactly what you don't want, as you have primed yourself for this.

For example, if you wish to cut out junk food, the correct phrasing would be, "I treat my body to healthy food", rather than, "I no longer enjoy fatty food and sweets."

Being detailed is also important. For example, "I feel wonderful eating bowls of yummy vegetables. I feel lighter and more energized, and my tummy feels less bloated." This is way more powerful than just saying, "I eat vegetables."

Keep it realistic. You won't lose all the weight overnight, you won't "always drink two liters of water", but you might say, "I hydrate whenever I think about it."

Attach positive feelings. Don't just say, "I am losing a pound a week." Rather, go for a more lively and energizing language, like "I am proud to be steadily losing weight."

Here are some examples for weight-management affirmations:

- I am trim, slim, and sexy.
- I nourish myself with healthy, delicious food.
- I am honoring my body.
- I am healthy and whole.
- It is easier each day to calm my mind and fall asleep faster.
- I am connected with my body's healing and recovery abilities.
- I am feeling more confident each day.
- I am more aware of my feelings and can guide them in a more positive direction.
- I am more at peace and at ease with myself.

Once you have your short-list of affirmations, you will use them as part of your self-hypnotherapy.

The other little trick is to create a weight-loss mantra. This can be taken from the most powerful affirmation you have created, or you can create a whole new statement. For me, a calming mantra was most important in the early days, but you can change these as you go. Examples of mantras could be: "I'm okay", "Every day, and in every way, I am getting better", "Let it be", or "I'm doing well."

When your day starts feeling tough and challenging, haul out your mantra and quietly repeat it to yourself.

Self-Hypnotherapy

Take your list of affirmations and write them up and stick them somewhere you will see right before bed, and after waking. You can also say them out loud at these times, or even right after meditation.

You can record them and use them during meditation, or as a background recording with some music, played softly on a timer as you fall asleep.

All of this helps your goals sink deeply into your subconscious, which can then support you in achieving your goals. It's the power of belief in yourself.

Mindful Eating

This is a method that can help you regain control over your eating in a gentle, yet focused manner. Based on Buddhist concepts, it is a form of meditation combined with the act of eating. Meditation is not about zoning out, but instead about becoming super focused and calm.

When we eat mindfully, we are paying full attention to the experience, our mental state, as well as to our body's feedback.

It is a holistic approach that we have already used extensively throughout this book. However, to fully appreciate the method, let's summarize it here.

First, it is about eating slowly, such as savoring every bite, being fully in the moment, and the action of eating from a sensory point of view. You fully engage with the colors, sounds, textures, shapes, smells, and flavors.

It is about eating without any other distractions, like the TV, a book, or your phone. These all take your focus off the eating experience and can mask what is happening in your mind and body, so it's best to remove them if you can.

Knowing, and being fully dialed into your body and its cues around hunger and fullness is the other part of it. It is eating only when truly hungry and knowing the difference between true hunger and an emotional trigger. So, this means being super aware of your inner state of being as much as possible. This also means stopping, or not eating, when your body doesn't need to.

When it comes to mindful eating, your overall focus is health and well-being, and not anything else. However, this does not mean that you don't give thanks for, and fully appreciate the bounty of food in front of you at a meal.

Lastly, mindful eating means removing the guilt, fear, boredom, and shame. This means dealing with these feelings separately from and using more constructive methods than eating to console and soothe yourself. If you become aware that bad feelings are triggering your current craving, use any of the tools I have given you to process the emotion in a healthy way.

Staying conscious of your inner world on a physical, emotional, and mental level is reinforced by actions like meditation, mindfulness, and focus exercises.

Part of the lead-up to a food addiction is that we have become automatic eaters. We eat what is put in front of us. We eat at certain times, regardless of how hungry we are, and we eat mindlessly as we watch the latest TV show, while working, reading, or playing computer games. How can we be tuned into our bodies in this way? We need to pay attention to our food and eating patterns. We need to slow down, and stop multitasking, which is one of the fundamental pleasures of life if we are to become more mindful of our actions.

Brain-Body Methods

Research has uncovered some super useful information about mood management recently. The consensus is that while dealing with your thoughts and cognitive processes are important, there are also quicker, more direct body-brain interventions that can help manage and reduce bad feelings quickly and effectively.

These are ways to calm, heal, and train your nervous system directly, and without having to think too much about it. This dials into our natural calming response, which works in opposition to our fight-freeze-flight response that activates us to deal with danger (Therapy in a Nutshell, 2021).

A healthy nervous system needs to be predominantly in a calm state, and only occasionally in a high-alert state. However, due to our modern-day lives that involve many perceived dangers and fears, we tend to stay in the high-alert fight-freeze-flight state way more than we should. The crazy traffic, our demanding boss, the stuff we see on the news, and that unpaid bill, all add up. Our brain reacts as much to these perceived threats as to real ones, and our systems stay flooded with adrenaline, cortisol, and other stress hormones. Over time, our brains become hardwired for stress, and we become more easily anxious, stressed, and hypervigilant. We startle or crack at the smallest things. We burn out, end up with full-blown panic attacks, and more.

To get past trauma and stress out of your body, and to regulate your nervous system quickly, consider one of these methods for fast relief. It's all about triggering our calm state as often as possible, as well as processing the stress chemicals out of our systems faster.

Shake and Dance it Off

Look at the work done by James Gordon, a trauma specialist who has worked with rape victims, war and disaster survivors, and many others traumatized in various ways. Most of these people were dealing with complex post-traumatic stress disorders by the time he got involved.

There is a particular case where he was running a workshop for survivors of a Haiti earthquake. He got them all shaking themselves about, and within a few minutes, a lot of emotion was released. After some crying among the 100-strong group of young women nurses, he got them all dancing to some Bob Marley. Many of the attendees reported that this was the first time since the trauma that they had been able to cry or laugh. They had been in a frozen emotional state and unable to process the terrible events. His shake therapy helped them break free way faster than many talk therapy sessions could have done (Therapy in a Nutshell, 2021).

So, give it a go. Stand comfortably, put on your favorite music if you want to, and start consciously shaking yourself around for a few minutes. Don't hurt yourself, obviously, just loosely shake each leg, arm, hand, foot, and your torso. The music helps as this method is a bit like dancing at a club if you think about it.

Then take a few minutes and do some deep breathing, or belly breathing, and then dance it off some more. Have fun with it. A few minutes of this should see your stress levels reduced.

If you've ever watched *Grey's Anatomy*, you will know all about how Grey and Yang use dance to destress and let go after a hectic day in the ER!

Move Quickly

At the first sign of distress, get moving as soon as you can. Whether you go for a brisk walk, do a few jumping jacks, twirl around, or go to the restroom and do a few calisthenics, just move. This works the stress chemicals out of your body and gives your body and brain a chance to calm down, and to heal from past continuous stress. You are teaching yourself to process and calm down on command almost.

Allow Emotions to Manifest

By this, I don't mean to take out your anger on people in a negative or harmful way. However, when you are in the grip of an emotion, find some sort of release that works for you.

Crying is one of our body's self-soothers, strangely enough. So, if you can allow yourself a good cry, do it. Try not to let your higher cognitive thinking interfere with all kinds of judgments. You can take yourself off somewhere private to do this if you need to. You may end up with a red nose and a bit of a headache, but you will feel the ease that comes from emotional release, too.

Channeling your emotions into some sort of activity helps. Household chores, that report you have been procrastinating, or that garden work that's piling up, are all great options. If you are an artistic type, painting, working with clay, or whatever materials you prefer can also be a release, as can writing about your feelings and the situation.

Sometimes, I will write it out, and then safely burn the result as a kind of mental and visual closure on the issue.

However, my point is to let yourself feel the feelings, and allow your natural physical reactions wherever you can, in a safe space, and in a way that is not harmful to anyone else or yourself.

Weight it Out

Using weighted blankets or piling on blankets and cushions can supply a level of warmth and comfort that could ease your need to go seeking it in junk food. Wrapping yourself like a burrito in blankies is also a great way to soothe yourself.

Acupressure and Acupuncture

Anecdotal evidence suggests that this can work to help lower stress levels and manage moods better. For acupuncture, you would need to find a trained therapist who understands how the body's energy works. Coincidentally and interestingly, the ancient Chinese art of acupuncture maps out these energy channels that we can now confirm match up to our nervous system.

For an at-home method, you can use acupressure on yourself. This is just gentle, firm pressure on specific spots, such as:

- Between your eyebrows.
- The top of your ear, where the ear curls over slightly, close to your head.
- The soft tissue between your index finger and thumb.
- On your inner arm, about three fingers width above your wrist.
- The spot where your neck ends, and your shoulder starts.
- On the top of your foot, in between the big toe and second toe.

Exercise that Works

While you can't exercise off much of those extra calories you ate earlier today, there are always benefits to a regular exercise program.

Exercise helps you regulate your mood, and for that around 20 to 30 minutes of medium-paced movement every day is sufficient. You also want to exercise for muscle toning, strength, and physical endurance. Resistance training and aerobic exercise can also help counter the loss of bone density and muscle, and this becomes vitally important, especially as we get older.

More importantly, exercise, when done regularly, helps increase your RMR (resting metabolic rate) and that means you burn more calories in general than if you didn't exercise. This certainly helps maintain a more consistent weight, too. Once you lose weight, exercise helps you keep it off.

The US Department of Health recommends about 150 minutes per week of moderate aerobic activity like brisk walking, swimming, brisk chores and gardening, dancing, or jogging. Strength exercises should be a minimum of twice a week and include a single set of exercises targeting each muscle group. You can use weight machines or equipment and basic calisthenics with rubber stretch bands, weights or just using your own body weight, like squats, arm, and leg lifts, planking, wall presses, pushups, pullups, sit-ups, and so on (Mayo Clinic, 2019).

There is evidence to show that certain types of exercise are more effective overall when it comes to weight management.

Walking is probably the best way for beginners to start building their fitness levels. It needs no equipment, and your steps can add up quickly. It's low impact, which is important, especially if your body and joints are already stressed by extra weight.

Swimming is very relaxing and grounding, and is low impact, while still being fairly aerobic. The butterfly stroke uses the most energy, followed by breaststroke and simply treading water. You could literally just go hang out in the pool with your besties for an hour, talking and treading water, and you would lose around 700 calories that way (Raman, 2019).

Other choice for faster weight loss is HIIT (high-intensity interval training). This technique means you burn more calories while spending less time doing so. You can choose any kind of exercise, as it is all in the intensity and duration. The idea is to exercise as hard and fast as you can for around 30 seconds, and then slow it down, but keep going for about a minute or two, then repeat. Keep going for 10 to 30 minutes, depending on your fitness level.

If you have not been exercising, I strongly recommend adding this in slowly, using the habit formula I gave you earlier in the book. However, taking a holistic look at your weight management plan and including as many elements as you can that will support you will ensure more consistent results in the long run. Lastly, it's advisable for you to have a chat with your doctor before you start any exercise program.

Chapter 9: Step 7—Set No More and Next Goals. Repeat!

To achieve anything in life, we need to be clear on what that is. A big reason why many people don't achieve their goals is that their goals are simply too vague. Moreover, they don't keep those goals clearly in mind, even if the goal has been well-defined, unless it is truly moving and inspiring for them.

The guy who vaguely thinks about having a social gathering with some of his best friends, but does not get clear on when, where, how, and who will attend, will definitely not be having that party. The person who swears vengeance on the criminal who abducted his family, as we see in the movies, is relentless in the pursuit of his goal. I know that movies are just fiction, but this example gives you an idea of the degree of commitment and passion you need to aim for. In the movie *Taken*, Liam Neeson was certainly not vague about what he wanted to achieve. It took some skills to get there, but even if he hadn't had those, I have the feeling that character would have never given up.

You need to get just as serious and clear about your weight management goals. You need to really get why they are important and keep this always front and present in your mind. The more positive emotion you can attach to these goals the better. Go back to my section on visualization and affirmations if you need a refresher.

Calculate your Calorie Target

Your calorie needs are decided by age, weight, height, lean body mass, gender, and level of activity during the day.

Have you worked out your own calories target yet? It can be pretty complex working it all out from scratch and there is no need. If you don't like math, just use an online calculator, like the NHS (UK's National Healthcare Service) BMI healthy weight calculator. Most of them are pretty accurate.

Set Your Food and Lifestyle Goals

With your daily calorie target in mind, and now knowing what you do about healthy eating, make yourself a list of foods, serving portions, and related calories.

It's best to choose foods that you know you enjoy, although without any of the junk foods, added sugars and fats. By choosing stuff you already like, keeping your healthy favorites readily available, and eating lots of that, within your calorie budget, it makes the whole process a lot easier.

What is important for this decision-making time is listing your lifestyle priorities, too.

Practical Exercise: Create a Healthy Living Visual

Create a visual reminder on a large piece of card or erasable board that you stick up in the kitchen or bathroom.

At the top, write your current calorie daily budget.

Underneath, list all the foods you like and that also classify as healthy. Create three columns. In the first column, list all the high fiber, high-water content foods with a low-calorie density. For example, fruits, vegetables, non-fat dairy, and whole grain bread, pasta, or rice. These are often 'free' foods that you can eat quite a lot of, and fill your plate and tummy up with, rather than any of the other options. In the second column, list the foods that are still healthy, but are slightly higher in calories, like fish, chicken, cooked beans, eggs, avocados, low-fat cheese, legumes, and hummus. These need to be monitored and limited to some degree. In the third column, list those foods that you like, but that are high-calorie density and only allowed in specific, small portions, like bacon, butter, red meat, dried fruit, nuts, oils, peanut butter, seeds, wine, and full-fat dairy. You could even write in the calorie amount for each food next to it if that makes your life easier.

This helps keep it present in your mind, whenever you reach for a bite.

Lastly, list your current lifestyle priority. This will be an area of your life that requires attention, and which is directly impacting your weight management. It could be sleep quality, activity levels, stress control, hydration, mindfulness, or whatever you feel you need right now more than all the others. Remember to pick one thing at a time. You know how habits work now, right? Your other option is, as we mentioned earlier, to habit bundle stuff, and then you can perhaps add more.

This does not mean you can't make a good effort to do all the other things, as and when you can, but your energy and focus is going on habituating only one major lifestyle change for now.

Therefore, I like to use an erasable board, because in a few weeks' time, my goal might progress to the next good habit, because I have the current one fully set, or I may discover new foods and tastes I can add to my food lists.

I do this in addition to my calorie-tracking apps on my phone.

No More and Next Goals

As part of an addiction prevention mindset, you need to be very clear on what you want and don't want to happen. Setting No More and Next goals are our last major step in the 3+4 Method journey.

Practical Exercise: No More and Next

Regular weigh-ins are an important part of helping you stay focused on your goals. You can expect your weight to sometimes be slightly more or less by around a pound, due to water retention or loss, and you can at times hit that weight plateau we mentioned before. However, what you want to see is a gradual decrease. This is where No More and Next goals work so well.

1. Weigh yourself regularly. Weekly, on the same day, at the same time, is a good idea.

2. Note your current weight and date.

3. Update your goals. The No More goal is the weight you don't want to gain ever again, and your Next goal is the weight you are aiming for. The Next goal should be a short-term goal and not the final goal weight that you want.

4. You can write your overall goal weight up if you want on your healthy living board next to your calorie budget.

The No More and Next goals are dynamic, periodically adjusted, based on your new weight. Be careful not to set unrealistic Next goals, because if you repeatedly don't make that goal, you may get demotivated.

The No More goal is as important as the Next goal. People generally focus on losing weight without putting all the effort into ensuring they will not gain [X] pounds of weight ever again.

When you achieve your Next goal, adjust the goalposts again. Although you may feel proud of yourself, be careful not to fall into the trap of celebration.

The key is understanding that losing weight is not about celebrating but adjusting your No More and Next goals. Forget about external factors, such as people telling you that you look great and thinner, that your clothes are big now, or that you feel you deserve a reward. Forget about it. This is about being logical. You are dealing with an addiction.

It sounds harsh, but simply update your No More and Next goals and move on.

Represent and Repurpose

Regularly remind yourself why you are doing what you are to control your weight. Whatever your values are, keep them front and center in your head.

You are not just beating an addiction. You are beating an addiction for a reason. What is that? Put that up on your vision board and healthy living board as well. Every morning and evening, quietly tell yourself, "I am doing this because..."

Actually, say it out loud, and even better, say it to yourself in the mirror. This makes it more personal and helps you feel stronger.

Constantly remind yourself about your struggles from steps 1 to 3 (Addiction, Long term goals, Stop believing you know it all), and fully commit to steps 4 to 7 (Extreme discipline, No Exceptions, Eating healthily, No More and Next goals), over and over again. Do this, and I assure you that you'll gain a healthy weight for life.

Chapter 10: Stay Mindful of Your Addiction

This is not just a weight-loss book, as you know. Too many of us are genuinely addicted to food, especially all the wrong kinds of food. We use cookies, cakes, frappes, cupcakes, burgers, pies, fries, chips, junk snacks, and sweets to stuff our emotions down and distract us from unhappy thoughts and feelings. We have grown used to using food to soothe ourselves and need it in the same way that an alcoholic needs booze.

While food is always going to be pleasurable, and it should be, we need to distinguish between eating out of emotional need and discomfort or boredom and eating simply because we are maintaining our bodies and relishing the joys of life.

It is so much harder for a food addict in some ways. With other addictions, you get to walk away from the substance completely, but we never get to walk away from food. We have to try to find a balance and maintain our self-discipline at extraordinary levels for the rest of our lives. Because like with any addict, the chance of slipping back into our addiction is very real.

However, we can take a leaf from alcohol and drug addicts' books and use some of their methods to help us stay focused and on track with our new healthy lifestyles.

12-Steps

The 12-steps program has been used successfully for all kinds of addictions. They are way more than just a once-off process, they are a guideline to a new way of life. The 12 steps as used by Alcoholics Anonymous, and many other addiction support programs, are listed below.

Here are the 12 Steps as defined by Alcoholics Anonymous:

1. We admitted we were powerless over alcohol—that our lives had become unmanageable.
2. Came to believe that a Power greater than ourselves could restore us to sanity.
3. Decided to turn our will and our lives over to the care of God as we understood Him.
4. Made a searching and fearless moral inventory of ourselves.
5. Admitted to God, to ourselves, and to another human being the exact nature of our wrongs.
6. Were entirely ready to have God remove all these defects of character.
7. Humbly asked Him to remove our shortcomings.
8. Made a list of persons we had harmed and became willing to make amends to them all.
9. Made direct amends to such people wherever possible, except when to do so would injure them or others.

10. Continued to take personal inventory and when we were wrong promptly admitted it.

11. Sought through prayer and meditation to improve our conscious contact with God as we understood Him, praying only for knowledge of His will for us and the power to carry that out.

12. Having had a spiritual awakening as the result of these steps, we tried to carry this message to alcoholics and to practice these principles in all our affairs.

    (AA, n.d.).

I have taken the steps as listed, minus most of the bad language, from Russel Brand's *Recovery* book. Having engaged with the 12 steps via various groups, this resonated the best with me, as being a powerful and helpful way to engage with the process. I have also added my own touches here and there—those things that worked and continue to work for me.

Step 1: Honesty!
"Are you a bit f*cked?" (Brand, 2018)

If you can't name it, you can't own it. Often, we have been enduring addiction for many years, and we may feel ashamed, guilty, or fearful of other people's reactions and level of understanding. We have tried countless diets, exercise plans, and lifestyle changes, but none of them stick, and we know, if we are honest with ourselves, that we do indeed have a food addiction problem. We are using food to try and soothe or solve other problems in our lives. If you have read this far, you will very clearly know by now whether this is true for you or not.

You first need to admit you are an addict. And then you need to admit you have had no power or control over your addiction. Only then can you start the journey of positive change and healing. Admitting that you feel powerless does not mean that you are weak. It means admitting that you are living with a disease that affects your brain. If you stay in denial, you cannot even begin to work on the problem. Your ongoing inability to control your eating is outward evidence that you have had no control on your own.

Step 2: Faith

"Could you not be f*cked?" (Brand, 2018)

Do you understand that you need to make changes? Do you accept that this means you need to do something different than before? Is this going to be easy? Can you use the same thinking, methods, and tools you have used in the past? Did they work? Of course, the answer is no.

Something has got to give. You need to attain a new level of thought and connect with your chosen greater power consciously and often.

What is a power greater than me? Could that be God, nature, your sponsor, your mother, your family, spirit, or the power of people joined together in this fight against addiction?

Describe what you believe this greater power to be. Think about it. Write it down.

This can also be anything or anyone that makes you aware of how insane things have been. You also need to accept that you will need to open yourself up to spirit, support, and accept healing.

You may have your doubts or prejudices about the words "greater power", but you are not limited by this if you become aware of these thoughts and spend some time questioning them. Can you accept that there might be something greater than you at work in the universe? Do you know any other people who accepted and applied this thinking in their lives who are happy, connected, and healed (or even healers themselves)? Is that what you would like in your life?

Step 3: Surrender

"Are you, on your own, going to 'unf*ck' yourself?" (Brand, 2018)

Have you tried anything that has worked? If anything did work, would you be here at this moment?

Are you unhappy, depressed, anxious, or suffering in some way? Do you have a low self-worth? Is doubt or perfectionism weakening you? Is it clear yet that your past plans did not work? Could you be open to new information, and new ideas that could help?

By surrendering resistance to what is, and recognizing that you alone, and all you know so far, hasn't been enough to recover, you surrender and open yourself up to outside help. By surrendering, you make a clear decision, and thus an action, too.

Brand says, "We are trapped in a way of 'being' that is not working. Here are some categories which will help us amend our perspective. We can usually identify the root of pain and spiritual discomfort within these areas."

- Pride (what I think you think about me)
- Self-esteem (what I think about myself)
- Personal relations (the script I give others)
- Sexual relations (as in personal relations, but pertaining to sex)
- Ambitions (what I want in life, my overall vision of my 'perfect' self)
- Security (what I need to survive)
- Finances (money and how it affects my feelings)

(Brand 2018)

Step 4: Self-Awareness and Soul Searching

"Write down all the things that are f*cking you up or have ever f*cked you up and don't lie or leave anything out." (Brand, 2018)

This is a tough step. You need to get to the root of your addiction. You need to see what the cause and effect of all your addictive behaviors have been in the past. You need to admit any harm you have done to yourself and others.

The questions you need to ask include:

- Where did I make a mistake?
- Where have I been selfish?
- Where was I dishonest?
- Where was I afraid?
- Where am I to blame, at fault, or just plain wrong?

(Brand, 2018)

Brand uses a table that you can download if you search for the free pdf of *Recovery* by Russel Brand. It's a series of worksheets that you can use as a guide, and that relate to these steps.

Self-awareness is tough at times. We have to face parts of ourselves that we don't always want to admit. A lot of the self-awareness exercises in this book will help support you through this process, too.

Step 5: Integrity!

"Honestly tell someone trustworthy about how f*cked you are." (Brand, 2018)

Taking ownership of everything you uncovered in steps 1 to 3 (Addiction, Long term goals, Stop believing you know it all), you need to speak aloud these truths. You need to share them both with your higher power, whoever or whatever that is, and with at least one other trusted person. This is normally your mentor or sponsor who is supporting you through the process. Whoever they are, they should have no investment or agenda other than to help you.

Words spoken out loud defuse the power that those things from the past hold over us. It makes it easier to forgive, take the lesson, and let it go.

You may need several conversations to cover it all. Make sure that when you do share, you are taking full responsibility for your actions and thoughts.

Step 6: Acceptance!

"Well, that's revealed a lot of f*cked up patterns. Do you want to stop it? Seriously?" (Brand, 2018)

See yourself as you are—exactly as you are, right now. See all your faults and flaws and accept them and open up our thinking. We can then process faulty thinking, unhelpful core beliefs, analyze payoffs and fears, and then let that go.

If you are willing to change, how will things get better? If you don't change, what could happen? Taking responsibility for your own healing is a big part of this. It is not up to anyone else but you. You can still seek help and support, but you are the one making the decisions.

Step 7: Humility!

"Are you willing to live in a new way that's not all about you and your previous f*cked up stuff?" (Brand, 2018)

You have to let go of pride. And you need to commit to creating positive changes. Asking for help, and allowing it, is a big part of this step.

Step 8: Willingness!

You need to be willing to make amends for any harm you have caused yourself or others with your addictive behavior. You need to get very clear on what you did that was harmful, what you should have done differently and who suffered because of your actions.

You may find, with food addiction, that this is mainly you. However, there will be fallout on family and friends, not so much as a result of you being overweight, but from the emotional baggage you were not dealing with and numbing with food.

Step 9: Forgiveness!

"Now apologize. Unless that would make things worse." (Brand, 2018)

Here is where you seek forgiveness for the harm and make what amends you can.

If we apologize in the right way, it works well and can be the beginning of healing for you and others, too. This is a great formula for an apology.

1. First, make sure you are sorry. There is no point apologizing if it is fake—it will just break down everyone's faith in you even more in the long run.

2. Ask if this is a good time, if the person can spare you a few minutes, and if they are in an okay headspace for this conversation. If the answer is no, ask when they feel this might be. If the answer is never, leave it there. Obviously, this is going to be of further harm to them and so you have to stop. To force an apology or difficult conversation on anyone is abusive.

3. Say "I'm sorry."

4. Explain that you know why what you did was unacceptable to them. This is to show you understand exactly what you did wrong. They may want to add their own perspective here, and you need to let them and be open to hearing it.

5. Explain what you will do differently going forward to avoid a repeat of the problem. Don't use the words "I will try", just commit to the change fully.

6. Ask if there is anything you can do for them to make amends. They may not want anything, or they may have something in mind. Whatever it is, be sure to follow through, unless it is physically impossible or harmful to you or others.

Remember—the best apology is always changed behavior!

Forgiveness is another story. You cannot force anyone to forgive you. You can only ask for that forgiveness through an authentic apology.

However, you need to apply the forgiveness process to yourself, too. You need to get clear that if you knew better, or had the ability before, you would have done better. However, now you are in a stronger space. You do know better, and so now can do better. Take the lesson, and let go of the past, because otherwise the shame will consume you and stop your progress.

Step 10: Maintenance

"Watch out for f*cked up thinking and behavior and be honest when it happens." (Brand, 2018)

What are you actively doing to manage your addiction? You need to make a daily personal inventory of your actions and thoughts. What is serving you and what is not? What has happened today that is a warning sign, and what action needs to be taken to head off your addiction re-emerging. If you mess up, apologize, and make amends, even if this is just to yourself.

Commit to a lifetime journey of personal healing and growth. There will be inevitable challenges, and you now have most of the tools you need to deal with them.

Journaling, support groups, your mentor, and daily reflection can all help with this step.

Step 11: Stay mindful and Conscious

"Stay connected to your new perspective." (Brand, 2018)

Using meditation or prayer, stay in contact with your own self-awareness, and with your spiritual connection. Keep growing through conscious self-awareness and reflection. Accept that there are many things you still do not know that you are not broken, and that you are becoming. Just like the caterpillar needs to dissolve into a gooey mess before it can become a butterfly, you need to break your thoughts, feelings, and actions down to their parts, face them, and then learn from them continuously.

Step 12: Service!

"Look at life less selfishly, be nice to everyone, help people if you can." (Brand, 2018)

Share what you have learned, and support others as needed. You reinforce your healing in this way. Helping lifts the spirit.

Is there any specific strength or skill you have that you can use to do so? And are you able to balance this step with all your other responsibilities, like work, family, self-care, relationships, and other commitments?

What is true is that you cannot work these steps alone, no matter what version you ascribe to. At the very least, find a trusted sponsor or mentor to walk them with you.

12-Step Alternatives

If 12 steps do not appeal to you, there are a few other programs you might consider.

Self-Management and Recovery Training (SMART Recovery) places emphasis on coping with cravings, using cognitive behavioral therapy and other techniques to heal and shift toward a better life. They recognize that addictive behaviors serve a purpose, helping people to cope with bad emotions and life's challenges, so they offer other, less destructive methods to use in place of the addiction. They teach coping skills that you will use for the rest of your life. Their 4-point program involves:

1. Building and maintaining the motivation to change. The main goals of humans are survival, happiness, and avoiding pain. Most addictive behaviors are linked to these goals. SMART creates awareness that addictive behaviors are only short-term fixes that stop you from achieving these goals long term.

2. Coping with your addiction urges and cravings.

3. Managing thoughts, feelings, choices, and actions effectively, without resorting to the addictive behavior patterns.

4. Living a balanced, happy, and healthy life.

(Hazelden Betty Ford Foundation, 2019)

Secular Organizations for Sobriety (SOS) and LifeRing Secular Recovery both take a non-spiritual approach based on cognitive therapy and other modalities which help an addict set up successful strategies.

Refuge Recovery is based on Buddhist principles that in themselves direct practitioners away from the physical reliance on and attachment to a substance or activity that causes suffering.

Whatever methods you choose to assist you on your journey to wellness, and in your fights against addiction, depend on what resonates with you.

This book, focused as it is on food addiction, combines many of the methods and modalities used by all these programs and combines them in one practical approach to the problem that has worked for me, and for many others I know.

Food addiction is a real thing. We need to sit up, open our eyes, and face the facts. Too many of us struggle with weight and are burdened with emotional issues, both linked to and underlying our eating choices. The advertising and marketing strategies of junk and fast-food companies have no regard for our health. We are surrounded by careless, and uncaring, temptation. So, we need to get real, admit the problem, and start taking the steps needed to turn our lives around.

Chapter 11: Addiction Strategies

We have come so far. By now, you understand the 3+4 Method well.

Step 1—Remind yourself you are an addict.

Step 2—Admit you struggle to commit to long term goals.

Step 3—Stop believing you know it all.

Step 4—Gain extreme discipline.

Step 5—Say No to exceptions.

Step 6—Eat healthily.

Step 7—Set No More and Next goals. Repeat!

However, what you may not yet have internalized is how to approach food addiction from an overall strategic point of view. Even though my steps take you very specifically through a tried-and-tested process, I want to make sure you truly understand what you are doing, and in what order, so your food addiction does not overwhelm you.

In the beginning of your food addiction recovery journey, your focus must not and cannot be on weight loss. I know that that is what is probably at the top of your mind and your priorities list, but a little patience is key to ultimate success.

If you really get that this is a food addiction, you need to take it seriously, and that means following the guidelines of the many therapists and recovered addicts like me. This is not a fad or a pop craze. Food addiction is a real mental disease. Increasingly, studies are proving that it is not just psychological, but also physically provable. MRI scans showing how the addiction-linked parts of the brain light up in overweight and food-addicted people as opposed to those with no food addiction. These tests are showing clear differences.

Think about it for a minute. Do you hear much about those people who binge on bowls of broccoli and apple? Or who overeats plates of pumpkin? Not really, right?

Why can some people buy a bag of cookies, or a pint of ice cream, and it lasts them the whole month, and others eat that in an hour? Those who eat it so fast probably only intended to have one cookie or one bowl of ice cream, but it backfired. This happened, because their reward centers in their brain, and their addiction, is in the driver's seat.

The addict feels satisfied, and yet also stuffed, perhaps ill, and probably also guilty or ashamed of their loss of control. However, those feelings won't stop it from happening again.

See, broccoli, and apples are not addictive. It's the sugars, salts, and fats that get us. High-fat, high-sugar, processed foods designed to max out our taste buds are what the real problem is, not the food itself.

If you start out trying to deal with the cravings and lose weight all at once, it becomes a nearly impossible endeavor.

So, the first step is spending at least a few weeks running through the self-awareness exercises I have given you in steps one through five (Addiction, Long term goals, Stop believing you know it all, Extreme Discipline, No Exceptions). During this time, consider also addressing at least one primary habit, and I would normally say choose between either sleep quality or exercise. At the same time, you can start putting other support systems in place, like finding a buddy or mentor, joining a support group, or finding a therapist who specializes in addiction.

When you feel ready, the next priority is to simply eat more healthily. Do not go on a diet! There is a reason why this book is titled, *Forget About Diets*. It's not just to be melodramatic. It's based on neuroscience, human behavior, and a thorough understanding of how food addiction works.

So, drop the diet fetish, even if you are compelled to try Paleo, Mediterranean, vegan, or any other apparently healthy diet, just leave it for now. You can do that later.

At first, you just want to get healthier, not thinner.

This will mean slowly swapping out the unhealthy foods for the healthier replacements. That's step six (Eat Healthily). However, currently, do not under any circumstances start weighing yourself, worrying about calorie counting, BMIs, or anything like that. All you want to do for the next month or so is swap out unhealthy for healthy. While you are doing what you can, continue with the self-awareness, self-growth, therapy, and other self-care habits in the order in which you have prioritized them.

It takes time for your body to get used to the new normal. Healthier eating also means that over time your cravings will lessen. Once your body is getting an optimal amount of nutrients in a form it can easily process, your brain also starts rewiring itself. Your opiate, or reward centers become less easily stimulated, and your insulin levels stabilize. This altogether means you have your addiction under far better control than when you began.

In the first few months, do not:

- Go on a diet.

- Eat high-sugar, high-fat, or processed foods. And you need to know that this change is forever. Once you have swapped a food out, stick with it until eventually all this stuff is gone from your meal choices.

- Obsess about your size or weight.

- Be afraid to say no, or to tell friends and family that you cannot eat something.

Do:

- Regain control of your eating habits. This is where your focus must be.

- Make eating and meal plans.

- Shop according to your plans.

- Get rid of junk food out of the house, fridge, and cupboard, if possible.

- Avoid junk food outlets altogether. If you must, take another route that does not take you past your favorite junk food outlets.

- Identify places, foods, events, and feelings that trigger your need to eat. Plan to deal with all of them.

- Always keep a healthy meal or snack on hand, and never let your hunger get above a 3 on a 1 to 5 scale where 5 is starving.

- Put support systems in place.

- Work on boundaries and saying no.

- Focus on healing past wounds and present suffering of any kind.

- Build your ability to focus through meditation and similar.
- Practice conscious self-awareness, and either work through the cognitive exercises I have given you, or get external help, or both.
- Share your goals with your trusted loved ones.

Food addiction is not taken as seriously as it should be. Most people battle to even understand drug or alcohol addiction, and these are painted with a dark and judgmental brush as it is. The words impulsive, out-of-control, wild, reckless, irresponsible, and so on are common to hear in relation to any addictive behavior. When it comes to food addiction, the general lack of understanding means that many people will not get that it is a real thing.

There is probably no real malicious intent, but you still need to deal with the fallout. The words lazy, greedy, and lack of self-control may be dropped around you like hurtful stones. Others may not understand the depth of your struggle. They may even be a part of the problem.

You will need to advocate for yourself and educate as much as possible. And you need to understand that their lack of knowledge, empathy, or comprehension is not your problem. This means growing a thick skin when people don't respond to your self-advocacy.

However, this will get easier, as you do the self-care work that heals your mind, heart, and soul. Each fear, bad memory, or bad feeling you face, and process, makes you that much stronger.

Only once you have the healthy eating and healthy mind down, and you feel confident that you have made sufficient progress in these areas, should you start looking at step 7 (No More and Next goals). That is when daily weigh-ins, calorie counting, and the No More and Next goals kick in.

By then, this will be much easier, and you may find that in the interim, you have lost some weight in any case, even though that wasn't your primary goal at first.

Medications for Food Addiction

If you are seeing a doctor or psychiatrist, they may also recommend medication to go along with whatever therapy you are having. They may suggest anti-anxiety, antidepressants, sleeping pills, and so on. Be sure to do your homework around what the different options are, how addictive they are, and how they may affect weight gain.

Weight-loss drugs, as we have discussed previously, don't really make a difference, because many of them are not that effective on their own, and don't address the root of the addiction.

Chapter 12: Stay Inspired

This is not about sharing endless personal stories about people who have made it. I find this type of thing only motivates you for a very short period, and unless the people I mention are personally known to you, it feels more like a fairy tale, and an impossible dream that only applies to other lucky people.

So, while I shared a bit of my own story, that is all you will see throughout this book.

By now you have had a lot of practical work and exercises that I strongly hope you have spent enough time with. If you skipped or skimped, now is a great time to go back and revisit all of them, especially with the new thinking you would have picked up by reading this far.

Sometimes, we need to revisit a concept many times. For me, it is like a spiral. You may keep going back to a particular idea or exercise and that's okay, because each time you come back with slightly higher awareness, and that always adds new learning to the mix. You might want to mark certain passages in the book that you can return to, to help you stay on track. Even though I wrote this book, I have also done that. I, too, need extra inspiration from time to time.

As an extra bonus, because we know we need all the help we can get, I have included a few extra strategies in this chapter, to help you stay inspired and motivated.

The Ulysses Pact

Ulysses was an incredibly ingenious hero during the ancient Trojan war. He was famous for his wily mind. Ulysses wanted to hear the famed Sirens' song, but he knew that this would make him incapable of rational thought. Sirens were known to lure men to their deaths on the harsh seas and rocks, with the beauty of their voices.

He made a pact with his men. He put wax in his men's ears to deafen them and had them tie him to the mast. He ordered them not to change course and to stop him if he should break free of his ropes.

When he heard the Sirens' song, Ulysses was driven momentarily insane and tried mightily to break free so that he might join the Sirens, which would have meant his death. His men kept the pact, and so Ulysses both heard the beguiling song, and kept his life.

This pact requires that you make a clear choice, now. Yes, even before we realize how hard things might get. However, that pact is an oath and binds you by your honor to stick to it, even when things do get hard later, as we know they will.

You can lock in your pact using one of your values. If it is the honor of your word, then it might be enough to give it to someone you highly respect. As we mentioned earlier, if you value money, give a friend a couple of checks that they can cash whenever you fail on your word.

The Seinfeld Strategy

This strategy comes from comedian Jerry Seinfeld, and I have personally used it and find it very useful in my weight-loss journey.

"He told me to get a big wall calendar that has a whole year on one page and hang it on a prominent wall. The next step was to get a big red magic marker.

He said for each day that I do my task of writing, I get to put a big red X over that day. After a few days, you'll have a chain. Just keep at it and the chain will grow longer every day. You'll like seeing that chain, especially when you get a few weeks under your belt. Your only job next is to not break the chain.

Don't break the chain,' he said again for emphasis." (Wignall, 2019)

You could use this to mark off each day that you meet your current goals, whether those are calorie intake, personal growth, No More and Next goals, movement, hydration, or any one of the many self-care and self-awareness habits I have already presented to you.

Never Forget Why

Always stay clear on what has driven you to make the changes you have chosen. It might be helpful to take some photographs of yourself as you are before you start your weight loss journey, and take measurements of your hips, buttocks, upper arms, belly, and thigh circumference.

Write a short list of exactly how you feel, and what events have occurred, that finally led you to the breakdown you needed to make a change. When you feel like giving up, take some new measurements, look at the old photos, and your list to remind you of the progress you have made.

Have Some Fun

Even though you may be deadly serious about turning your food addiction around once and for all, this does not mean that you can't also laugh a little and enjoy yourself.

In fact, a sense of humor, and laughter, are so extremely good for you that I recommend them every day. Doctor's orders!

You may need to get a little creative, but there are a few ways I can suggest:

- Use crazy dancing or join a movement class that you know you suck at.
- Add some music to any activity you are doing, even if it is just washing the dishes.
- Race against time. See who can drink their glass of water faster or walk around the block in record time. It helps to have another person involved. Otherwise, you can create your own time sprints and keep records.
- Celebrate, without food. For instance, enjoy family movie nights, explore new places or sites of interest, or perhaps reward yourself with an item you have been wanting, like a new book, or that Fitbit watch.

- Create ritualized fun. Make a big deal about laying the table, putting out candles, and playing ambient music, before your dinner, even if you are eating alone. Perhaps even dress up. These are things that our grandparents did as a matter of course, not because they were stuffy and boring, but because it was fun to do.
- Do stuff together with others. Unless you really are a complete introvert, and even then, I will bet you can find at least one person who might do for fun company while you exercise or pursue many other of your self-care goals.

Keep Learning

Whether you read, or watch YouTube videos, or join a master class online, just keep learning stuff.

I like to pick subjects related to whatever my current challenge is, or to a challenge of someone that I know or am trying to help. I surf the internet, watch TED talks, grab a book from the 2nd-hand shop or library, and indulge in feeding my brain, and not my body.

It just takes one little sentence or idea to springboard new inspiration and excitement for you.

Share

Consider creating a blog about your journey and challenges, or about any topic that interests you. Sharing your weight loss with others can be hugely motivational for you on several levels. Not only do you feel good for sharing your progress, but it also adds as an extra motivator, because you don't want to let your audience down by slipping up. To avoid that pain, you tend to stay more self-disciplined, too.

Create a Success and Gratitude Journal

Every day list a few things you got right, and a few things that you are grateful for. This helps keep your focus on the positive stuff and keeps you positively inspired, too.

Create a Competition

If you are doing this weight-loss thing with friends and family, create some goals and see who gets there first.

You obviously don't all have the same weight goals, but you can set markers that equate to each other up front and compete on things like how many fruits and veggies you eat, how much water you drink, or how much extra movement you manage in a day.

Set a fun reward for the winner that does not involve food, or if it does, let it be a voucher to a health food store.

Plan Your Daily Goals

You can add this to your healthy living board, or wherever you want. Just write up your top three goals for the day, first thing in the morning. What is crucial to do for you to feel you have met your healthy living goals, or at least made some progress?

Watch Some Movies

Yeah, I know other people's stories aren't always the answer, however, it can help uplift you when you are feeling a bit down.

Some great uplifting stories about weight loss, and resilience, or both, include:

- GI Jane
- Super Size Me
- Run Fatboy Run
- Center Stage
- The Pursuit of Happiness
- Unbroken
- Disfigured
- The Vicar of Dibley
- Shallow Hal

- Heavy Weights
- Precious
- Fat

All you need to do is search for movie lists with suggestions targeting the life issue you want a bit of inspiration with. Try it.

Stick it Up

I like to stick up inspirational quotes in my bathroom. It's a bit obvious, but it helps me when I'm going through a rough time, and I also use it to help my family, too, if I notice there is an issue they are struggling with.

I make sure to change the printouts regularly, because after a while, you truly stop seeing it, if you see it every day. You can find loads of memes, quotes, and similar on the internet.

Some of the quotes that have helped me in the past include:

"We become what we think about." —Earl Nightingale

"Happiness is not something readymade. It comes from your own actions." —Dalai Lama

"Success is not final, failure is not fatal: it is the courage to continue that counts." —Winston Churchill

"Believe you can and you're halfway there." —Theodore Roosevelt

"Move out of your comfort zone. You can only grow if you are willing to feel awkward and uncomfortable when you try something new." —Brian Tracy

"Everything you've ever wanted is on the other side of fear." —George Addair

"Your life only gets better when you get better." —Brian Tracy

"Happiness is not by chance, but by choice." —Jim Rohn

"If I cannot do great things, I can do small things in a great way." —Martin Luther King, Jr.

"We generate fears while we sit. We overcome them by action." —Dr. Henry Link

"We may encounter many defeats, but we must not be defeated." —Maya Angelou

"You are the sum total of everything you've ever seen, heard, eaten, smelled, been told, forgot—it is all there. Everything influences each of us, and because of that I try to make sure that my experiences are positive." —Maya Angelou

"There are no limits to what you can accomplish, except the limits you place on your own thinking." —Brian Tracy

"It's not whether you get knocked down, it is whether you get back up." —Vince Lombardi

Those are way more than you need to get started, but they have made a difference to me, in my journey. Take some time and go find ones that resonate with you. Stick them up and let them sink in over time.

Raising a Generation of Healthy Eaters

If you have children, it will very likely be on your mind that if you have a food addiction, they very well may also be potentially at risk. As many parents know, we manage to pay way more attention to the care of our children than we do to that of ourselves.

Everything you have learned about self-awareness, and healthy eating, can be equally taught to the next generation. More than likely, as you model good eating behaviors, your children will be watching and learning.

So, to help them, you need to help yourself first. This in itself can be very inspirational and motivating. Where we might battle to get a thing done for ourselves, we find extra energy to do the right thing for our children.

Wherever you are in your journey and no matter what age your children are, you may want to consider how you approach the whole concept of food with your children, to do your best to support them in their lifelong health needs, too.

Keep the conversation open. Talk often about why you are choosing certain foods over others, and why they are healthier. If your children are old enough, encourage them to do their own research, too. If they are still babies, you are in the lucky position of being able to set up good habits with them from the start, rather than trying to change bad habits that are already ingrained.

A few things to keep in mind are:

1. Steer clear of the empty-plate club. If a child has had enough to eat, do not force them to clear their plate.

This is not about you, or how long you spent slaving away over the meal. A clean plate does not necessarily mean a healthy child. Let them learn from an early age to listen to their own body's hunger cues, and to eat when hungry and stop when they are not.

2. Keep mealtimes distraction free. Remove tablets, TV screens and the like. If you can all sit down as a family to eat, all the better, but otherwise, make it a habit that they sit at a table and practice mindful eating for the time period appropriate for their age. Under eight years, if they can't sit still for long periods, allow them to excuse themselves from the table. A two-year-old can focus on eating for around six minutes, four years and they can go up to 12 minutes; eight-year-olds can be reasonably expected to sit at a dinner table for around 20 minutes; and 10-year-olds for around half an hour at the most.

3. Keep mealtimes light and calm. If they won't eat, don't make a big deal about it.

4. Offer a wide variety of healthy foods, and make sure you have healthy snacks available that they can help themselves to when they feel the need. A bowl of fruit that they can reach, or a snack plate with crudité, healthy dips like hummus and cottage cheese, cheese cubes, lean proteins, hard-boiled eggs, and so on that they can graze off when hunger hits ensures that they are getting enough food, and also enough of a variety of nutrients.

5. Let them eat with other kids. Often, children will try new foods, just because the other children are also eating it.

6. Encourage drinking water rather than fruit juices. If you are concerned that they aren't getting enough fruit or vegetables, offering smoothies and juices in between meals is fine (once they are weaned), but not a great idea right before a meal you would like them to eat. Those little tummies fill up fast on liquids, and then later when the rest of the family is finished eating, suddenly they are hungry.

7. Cook, prepare snacks, and shop together. You can teach them how to choose and prepare healthy meals this way, and use it as a teachable moment for budgeting, too.

Remember that everything you do and say is observed and learned from. It's not so much what you tell children to do, but what you model through your everyday behavior that will be the pivotal reason that they also learn healthier eating patterns.

By using your children as your reason to stay on track and focused on your own improved food choices, this can become a powerful driver of your own changed behavior, too.

Conclusion

There are more than 70 million food addicts in the United States alone: 50-percent of obese people, 30-percent of the overweight, and about 20-percent of those considered to be at a healthy weight who are really addicted to specific foods or amounts of food. There are around 400,000 deaths a year in the US that are obesity-linked. The estimated cost of extra medical care, lost workdays, and death, because of obesity, sat at about $117 billion in 2000 (Addiction Hope, n.d.). Twenty-plus years later, I am sure this has increased exponentially.

Why do we sit with such an endemic problem?

The definition of healthy eating is a confusing one. There are too many people out there trying to make money out of a life-and-death situation. Supermarket chains, fast-food outlets, diet gurus with "the answer", diet products like pills and supplements, all push their own agenda. Well, not all, but there is enough to muddy the water.

There is a smorgasbord of highly processed, cheap, and easy-to-access foods surrounding us on a daily basis. They are on every street corner, in every checkout queue, and sometimes even in schools. They are on social media, in media advertisements, and on billboards. They are packaged and presented in the most seductive ways imaginable. They are even offered to us lovingly and unconsciously by friends and family. These foods are high in sugar, additives, and unhealthy fats. And they are everywhere. They ring food addicts' pleasure centers like nothing else. The neural and physical rewards are extremely powerful and hard to resist.

And then we have our poor, abused bodies. They have not changed processes in countless centuries. They have no clue what to do with the modern-day food we fling down our throats. They have not yet adapted to the fast-food craze of the past 100 years. They store all the added, unnatural chemicals in our fat, and get confused by the sugars. We digest processed food so fast that we remain hungry and then eat more. This is mainly because the low-fiber content means that our stomachs don't get a chance to fill up enough to signal satiety.

The problem is that diets high in sugar and fats age us faster, mess with our brain function and, of course, make us gain weight, which has all the other health risks attached. Sugar ages your arteries, and saturated or trans fats contribute to various cancers. Not only do your arteries age, and your neurons get all inflamed, which leads to lack of focus, memory loss, and basically all the stuff brains do, not happening as well as it should, but it also ages your skin prematurely, too (WebMD, 2004). Want to look good into your old age? Well, then you know what you need to do.

Our education systems have, mostly, woken up to the fact that children need the facts, and we can find many life skills programs in schools now, although perhaps there is still not enough focus on self-awareness and dealing with the underlying issues that cause addictions in the first place.

Added to this, we have previous generations who endured incredible lack and deprivation during the last century. The world wars and various economic recessions created a certain kind of mentality that pushes clean plates and no waste.

Then we get our fast-paced lives, racing from home, school runs, and chores, to workplaces that put increasing pressure on us to produce, back to school runs, other commitments, childcare, relationships, and more. Perhaps we even try to fit some self-care, like the occasional gym session or a good night's sleep, in there. However, at times, we feel like we just never stop. The thought of adding extra work by cooking home-cooked meals, shopping healthily, and engaging with emotions and thoughts we may have been avoiding for decades, is probably too much to bear. It is easier just to grab dinner from a take-out place and tell ourselves we are doing our best.

You should be clear by now that you are an addict, and that to lose weight, you need to approach the problem differently. However, if you have any hesitation, go back over the signs.

- Do you eat when you are mad, sad, bored, or just because the food is there?
- Have you experienced significant weight gain?
- Do you often eat so much that you feel stuffed?
- Do you eat in secret, or try to hide your eating?
- Do you make a special effort to get your hands on certain foods, and are these foods high in fat or sugar?
- Do you eat so much that you feel sick?
- Do you suffer from joint pain, heart issues, high blood pressure, digestive problems, and inflammation because of your weight gain?
- Do you keep telling yourself you will sort this out, but you never do?
- Is there past trauma in your life, or unhappy thoughts and feelings, that you are afraid to face?
- Are you often anxious, stressed, depressed, angry, fearful, worried, ashamed, or irritable?
- Are your activities limited by your weight and fitness levels?

Any of these signs, especially linked to food and weight gain, are clearly pointing at food addiction.

The physical effects of food addiction include chronic pain, digestive issues, gut inflammation, reduced sex drive, headaches, obesity or unhealthy weight gain, diabetes, malnutrition, sleep issues, lethargy, arthritis, osteoporosis, and heart problems. The psychological effects include further depression, shame, low self-esteem, hopelessness, despair, and emotional dysregulation. And socially you can expect poor school or work performance, frequent sick leave days, isolation, family divisions and conflicts, a decrease in hobbies or interests, avoidance of social events, and financial difficulties because of some of this.

Is this the life you want for yourself? I strongly doubt it.

However, we need to eat. We cannot turn away from food in the same way an alcoholic turns away from alcohol, or a drug addict stops drugs. We have to fuel our bodies, or we die. So, we need to find a careful, self-disciplined, and conscious balance, and we need to recognize that we may tread this fine line for the rest of our lives. Addictions don't just disappear because our behavior changes. Even if we heal our trauma, shift our thinking, and have all our coping strategies and tools in hand, we can still slide back into full addiction if we are not alert and prepared.

Some people will argue that food can't be addictive because it is something we need to have. However, we don't really need all that high-fat, high-sugar, processed stuff, do we? While we may not get intoxicated, and there is no clear disruption of our daily lives, if we are addicted to the food, we are still addicts and need to take this very seriously.

People get that alcohol, drugs, cigarettes, or coffee can be addictive, but they haven't made the mental leap to the fact that the artificially occurring substances in processed food are just as bad, and just as reactive with our brains' reward centers. These substances fulfill every criterion for an addictive substance.

For instance, beef, cheese, meat, chocolate, and sugar are high on the addictive foods list in the diets of many Americans, according to Neal Barnard, the doctor who wrote *Breaking the Food Seduction*. The chemical compounds in high-fat, high-sugar, processed foods stimulate the brain's opiate and reward centers in such a powerful way that we literally cannot control our addiction. Unless we admit it and get the help we need.

Can you face it? Because only once you can admit to it, can you start fixing it.

The good news is that while we will perhaps have to stay conscious and disciplined for the rest of our lives, there are many ways to make this process a lot easier.

Losing weight consistently and permanently is not about fancy diets or a glamorous journey, but an arduous and tough path that requires discipline, commitment, and to stick with the 3+4 Method.

At first, you will need to engage with as many of the tools and strategies in this book as possible. You will need to do the work on a physical, mental, emotional, and self-care level. Each new choice will feel uncomfortable and a bit awkward, but if you stick with it, especially using our strategies for setting new habits, you will find your progress starts speeding up and it all gets a lot easier.

I have grown so much personally in this process. I am not afraid to admit that I was a food addict. I move through life, aware of my emotions. When they start signaling something is wrong, I listen to them and dig down to see what thoughts or contexts are creating this inner conflict. I have the tools to do so, and now so do you.

The idea of self-discipline no longer makes me think of people in camo gear doing push-ups until they crack. I see my extreme self-discipline as a guideline and a matrix within which I can be freer than ever before. It has become effortless and spilled over naturally into all other areas of my life. How else do you think I wrote this book? Sitting down to write every day takes focus and persistence, and that was easier, because I had already learned it during my food addiction journey.

Let's recap my main method.

The 3+4 Method states:

- Step 1—Remind yourself you are an addict.
- Step 2—Admit you struggle to commit to long term goals.
- Step 3—Stop believing you know it all.
- Step 4—Gain extreme discipline.
- Step 5—Say No to exceptions.
- Step 6—Eat healthily.
- Step 7—Set No More and Next goals. Repeat!

Over time, as you get used to the 3+4 Method, you will automatically do it.

Healthy food will be tastier than ever before. You will start seeing the physical and psychological benefits grow and have positive knock-on effects on the rest of your life, too.

It is not going to be quick, or easy. However, if you can persist, eventually it will stop taking up so much of your energy, and you will be able to focus on other priorities in your life while the 3+4 Method is working on autopilot.

Dealing with your food addiction will get easier. It starts with the first step, and then another, and another. Just keep going. Keep beginning again if you must, just don't ever give up. Success is possible. I and many other recovered food addicts are living proof of this. Use our lessons to help you on your way to a better life.

I believe in me, and I believe in you. The greater power of our collective efforts to support each other can create momentum and awareness worldwide. The growth of global consciousness around mental and physical health is a huge and gathering force. If I were a fast-food chain, or a food manufacturer or distributor, I would read the signs. Sooner than you think, they will either have to clean up their act or go out of business. Already, many governments are taking a sterner hand in passing laws around added fats and sugars.

The internet teems with self-help videos and content, all with the purpose of uplifting humanity and healing cycles of pain and suffering. Healing and health on all levels is the new social focus.

This is all so heartening.

Not to mention, the learning you have now, that will hopefully help you, and help anyone around you as you share what you have learned. Each small act of help and sharing creates positive ripples, and you can all make a difference. Whether it is through your buying choices, or through helping grow awareness of self-care, mental and emotional hygiene, or healthier eating choices.

Perhaps in our children's time, or their children's day, food addiction will only be a memory.

References

"6 Science-Based Health Benefits of Eating Vegan." *Healthline*, 23 Sept. 2016, www.healthline.com/nutrition/vegan-diet-benefits#TOC_TITLE_HDR_3.

"7 Powerful Strategies for Reaching Your Long Term Goals—RescueTime." *RescueTime Blog*, 3 Feb. 2021, blog.rescuetime.com/mental-strategies-long-term-goals. Accessed 17 Sept. 2021.

"10 Psychological Tricks to Stay Motivated and Stick with Your Goals." *Nick Wignall*, 8 July 2019, nickwignall.com/stay-motivated/.

"12 Step Recovery Programs Are a Guide for New Addiction-Free Lives." *Verywell Mind*, www.verywellmind.com/the-twelve-steps-63284.

Camille Noe Pagán. "Medications to Treat Binge Eating Disorder." *WebMD*, WebMD, 22 Jan. 2015, www.webmd.com/mental-health/eating-disorders/binge-eating-disorder/medications-binge-eating-disorder.

Centers for Disease Control and Prevention. "The Health Effects of Overweight and Obesity." *Centers for Disease Control and Prevention*, 17 Sept. 2020, www.cdc.gov/healthyweight/effects/index.html.

Davidson, Katey. "Mood Food: 9 Foods That Can Really Boost Your Spirits." *Healthline*, 5 Feb. 2020, www.healthline.com/nutrition/mood-food.

Dingemans, A. "Binge or Control? Assessment of the Validity, Treatment and Underlying Mechanisms of Binge Eating Disorder." *Scholarlypublications.universiteitleiden.nl*, 9 June 2009, scholarlypublications.universiteitleiden.nl/handle/1887/13829. Accessed 17 Sept. 2021.

"Does Sleep Affect Weight Loss?" *WebMD*, www.webmd.com/diet/sleep-and-weight-loss#1.

"Food Addiction Symptoms, Abuse Stats, & Side Effects." *Addiction Hope*, www.addictionhope.com/food-3/.

"Food Addiction: Craving the Truth about Food | Andrew Becker | TEDxUWGreenBay." *www.youtube.com*,www.youtube.com/watch?v=CopLIjQG1q0&ab_channel=TEDxTalk. Accessed 1 Aug. 2021.

Gunnars, Kris. "Top 12 Biggest Myths about Weight Loss." *Healthline*, Healthline Media, 3 July 2019, www.healthline.com/nutrition/top-12-biggest-myths-about-weight-loss.

"Harris-Benedict Calculator—Omni." *Www.omnicalculator.com*, www.omnicalculator.com/health/bmr-harris-benedict-equation.

"How Can I Burn 500 Calories in an Hour?" *MedicineNet*, www.medicinenet.com/how_can_i_burn_500_calories_in_an_hour/article.htm. Accessed 17 Sept. 2021.

"How Can I Burn 500 Calories in an Hour?" *MedicineNet*, www.medicinenet.com/how_can_i_burn_500_calories_in_an_hour/article.htm.

"How to Achieve 1 Pound of Weight Loss | Everyday Health." *EverydayHealth.com*, www.everydayhealth.com/weight/how-to-achieve-one-pound-of-weight-loss.aspx.

"How to Break Food Addictions." *WebMD*, www.webmd.com/food-recipes/features/breaking-food-adictions.

"How to Release Emotions Trapped in Your Body 10/30 How to Process Emotions like Trauma and Anxiety." *Www.youtube.com*, www.youtube.com/watch?v=GZw8fRPK-8k&ab_channel=TherapyinaNutshell.

https://www.facebook.com/NIHAging. "Serving and Portion Sizes: How Much Should I Eat?" *National Institute on Aging*, 2017, www.nia.nih.gov/health/serving-and-portion-sizes-how-much-should-i-eat.

https://www.facebook.com/verywell. "Using the Harris-Benedict Formula for Calculating Daily Calorie Intake." *Verywell Fit*, 2019, www.verywellfit.com/how-many-calories-do-i-need-each-day-2506873.

July 28, Lauren Brown West-Rosenthal, and 2016. "I Added This One Ingredient to My Water and My Cellulite Went Away." *Eat This Not That*, 28 July 2016, www.eatthis.com/essential-oils-weight-loss/. Accessed 17 Sept. 2021.

Kubala, Jillian. "12 Over-The-Counter Appetite Suppressants Reviewed." *Healthline*, Healthline Media, 25 Sept. 2018, www.healthline.com/nutrition/appetite-suppressants.

Mayo Clinic. "How Much Water Do You Need to Stay Healthy?" *Mayo Clinic*, 14 Oct. 2020, www.mayoclinic.org/healthy-lifestyle/nutrition-and-healthy-eating/in-depth/water/art-20044256#:~:text=The%20U.S.%20National%20Academies%20of.

MD, Robert H. Shmerling. "When Dieting Doesn't Work." *Harvard Health Blog*, 25 May 2020, www.health.harvard.edu/blog/when-dieting-doesnt-work-2020052519889.

"Motivation vs Discipline: The Yin and Yang of Health | Second Nature Guides." *Www.secondnature.io*, www.secondnature.io/us/guides/mind/motivation/motivation-vs-discipline.

NHS Choices. "Eat Well." *NHS*, 2 Aug. 2018, www.nhs.uk/live-well/eat-well/the-vegan-diet/.

"Office of Dietary Supplements—Omega-3 Fatty Acids." *Nih.gov*, 2017, ods.od.nih.gov/factsheets/Omega3FattyAcids-Consumer/.

"Psychedelic Therapy: Uses, How It's Done, Risks, and More." *Healthline*, 26 May 2021, www.healthline.com/health/mental-health/psychedelic-therapy#:~:text=Psychedelic%20therapy%20(sometimes%20referred%20to. Accessed 17 Sept. 2021.

Raman, Ryan. "The 8 Best Exercises for Weight Loss." *Healthline*, Healthline Media, 19 Aug. 2019, www.healthline.com/nutrition/best-exercise-for-weight-loss.

"Read Your Labels: 10 Harmful Food Additives to Avoid." *Www.acefitness.org*, www.acefitness.org/education-and-resources/lifestyle/blog/3188/read-your-labels-10-harmful-food-additives-to-avoid/. Accessed 17 Sept. 2021.

Sicat, Jeffrey. "Obesity and Genetics—Obesity Medicine Association." *Obesity Medicine Association*, 14 May 2019, obesitymedicine.org/obesity-and-genetics/.

"Sleeping Pills: The Pros and Cons." *WebMD*, www.webmd.com/sleep-disorders/features/sleeping-pills-pros-cons. Accessed 17 Sept. 2021.

"The 4 Phases of Weight Loss." *LIFT and LIVE FITNESS*, www.liftandlivefitness.com/nutrition/the-4-phases-of-weight-loss/. Accessed 17 Sept. 2021.

"The 4 Safest Sugar Substitutes and a Few to Avoid Completely." *Nutrition Action*, 20 June 2015, www.nutritionaction.com/daily/sugar-in-food/sugar-in-food-which-sweeteners-are-the-safest-and-which-should-you-avoid/#:~:text=The%20best%20and%20safest%20sugar. Accessed 17 Sept. 2021.

"The Science of Depression." *Www.youtube.com*, www.youtube.com/watch?v=GOK1tKFFIQI&ab_channel=AsapSCIENCE.

"The Twelve Steps of Alcoholics Anonymous." *Hazeldenbettyford.org*, 2019, www.hazeldenbettyford.org/articles/twelve-steps-of-alcoholics-anonymous.

"Throw Your Calorie Counter Away | Calorie Density." *Pritikin Weight Loss Resort*, 7 Nov. 2013, www.pritikin.com/your-health/health-benefits/healthy-weight-loss/1318-why-not-just-count-calories.html. Accessed 17 Sept. 2021.

"Top 10 Food Additives to Avoid." *Foodmatters.tv*, www.foodmatters.com/article/top-10-food-additives-to-avoid.

"What 500 Calories Really Looks like in Different Foods." *Lifehack*, 5 Aug. 2013, www.lifehack.org/articles/lifestyle/what-500-calories-really-looks-like-different-foods.html. Accessed 17 Sept. 2021.

"What to Know before You Buy Weight-Loss Pills." *Mayo Clinic*, 2018, www.mayoclinic.org/healthy-lifestyle/weight-loss/in-depth/weight-loss/art-20046409.

"Why Long Term Goals Don't Work and Short Term Goals Get Results." *Glasscubes*, 2016, www.glasscubes.com/why-long-term-goals-don-t-work-but-short-term-goals-drive-results/.

Printed in Great Britain
by Amazon

27584217R00128